FNA Cytology in the Diagnosis of Lymphoma

Monographs in
Clinical Cytology

Vol. 18

Series Editor

Svante R. Orell Kent Town

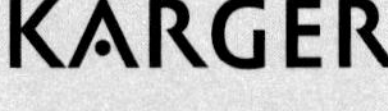

FNA Cytology in the Diagnosis of Lymphoma

Lambert Skoog Stockholm
Edneia Tani Stockholm

In collaboration with

Anja Porwit Stockholm

66 figures, 65 in color, and 8 tables, 2009

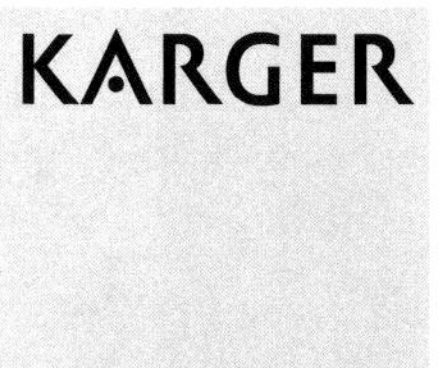

Basel · Freiburg · Paris · London · New York · Bangalore ·
Bangkok · Shanghai · Singapore · Tokyo · Sydney

··

FNA Cytology in the Diagnosis of Lymphoma

Lambert Skoog MD, PhD, Professor of Clinical Cytology
EdneiaTani MD, PhD, Associate Professor
Department of Pathology and Cytology
Karolinska University Hospital Solna
SE–171 76 Stockholm (Sweden)
Tel. +46 8 517 74525, Fax +46 8 517 74524
edneia.tani@ki.se
lambert.skoog@ki.se

Library of Congress Cataloging-in-Publication Data

Skoog, Lambert.
FNA cytology in the diagnosis of lymphoma / Lambert Skoog, Edneia Tani ; in
collaboration with Anja Porwit.
p. ; cm. -- (Monographs in clinical cytology, ISSN 0077-0809 ; v. 18)
Includes bibliographical references and index.
ISBN 978-3-8055-8626-9 (hard cover : alk. paper)
1. Lymphomas--Cytodiagnosis.   2. Needle biopsy.   I. Tani, Edneia.   II. Porwit,
Anja.   III. Title.   IV. Series.
[DNLM: 1. Lymphoma--pathology.   2. Biopsy, Fine-Needle. W1 MO567KF v.18 2008
/ QZ 350 S628f 2008]
RC280.L9S58 2009
616.4′207582--dc22
2008022915

Bibliographic Indices. This publication is listed in bibliographic services, including Current Contents® and PubMed/MEDLINE.

Disclaimer. The statements, opinions and data contained in this publication are solely those of the individual authors and contributors and not of the publisher and the editor(s). The appearance of advertisements in the book is not a warranty, endorsement, or approval of the products or services advertised or of their effectiveness, quality or safety. The publisher and the editor(s) disclaim responsibility for any injury to persons or property resulting from any ideas, methods, instructions or products referred to in the content or advertisements.

Drug Dosage. The authors and the publisher have exerted every effort to ensure that drug selection and dosage set forth in this text are in accord with current recommendations and practice at the time of publication. However, in view of ongoing research, changes in government regulations, and the constant flow of information relating to drug therapy and drug reactions, the reader is urged to check the package insert for each drug for any change in indications and dosage and for added warnings and precautions. This is particularly important when the recommended agent is a new and/or infrequently employed drug.

© Copyright 2009 by S. Karger AG,
P.O. Box, CH–4009 Basel (Switzerland)
Printed in Switzerland on acid-free and non-aging paper (ISO 9706) by Reinhardt Druck, Basel
www.karger.com
ISSN 0077–0809
ISBN 978–3–8055–8626–9

Contents

Contents

Acknowledgements

The completion of this book would not have been possible without the direct and indirect support and help from many individuals.

First, Drs. Sixten Franzén and Torsten Löwhagen, two pioneers who devoted their professional life to develop and spread the art of fine needle aspiration cytology. They were our mentors and friends who, with great enthusiasm and patience, shared their experience and ideas about fine needle aspiration cytology, in particular in the diagnosis of lymphoma.

We wish to express our deep appreciation to our friends Professors Mario Rubens Montenegro and Marcello Fabiano de Franco, Brazil, who encouraged one of us (E.T.) throughout the training in pathology and to go to the Karolinska Hospital for training in cytopathology. They represent the best blend of practical and academic pathology.

Professor Peter Biberfeld generously shared his vast experience of immunohistochemistry which allowed us to apply the technique to cytologic material. In this process and throughout the years, C.T. Margot Carlsson has provided invaluable assistance. Further, the expert secretarial help of Mrs. Margareta von Lampe is gratefully acknowledged.

Special thanks go to Professor Anja Porwit who established a center of excellence for flow cytometry at Karolinska Hospital and her expert contribution in chapter 3.

The contributions by Drs. Elisabeth Blennow, Jean-Louis Dargent and Veli Söderlund are gratefully acknowledged.

Without the financial support from the Cancer Society Stockholm and Magnus Nasiells fund, parts of our studies could not have been completed.

The continuous support and help provided by Dr. Svante Orell, the Editor of this series, and the staff of Karger Publishers contributed immeasurably to the completion of this book.

Preface

The enlarged lymph node became one of the main targets for fine-needle aspiration (FNA) cytology, and was soon accepted in the diagnosis of various types of lymphadenitis and metastatic disease. The diagnosis of lymphoma by FNA cytology was, however, controversial for many years in spite of early reports, in particular by Lopes Cardoso, which demonstrated the great potential of the technique. The scepticism at that time mainly resulted from the emphasis on growth patterns in the diagnosis and subtyping of lymphomas, Obviously, the growth pattern cannot be discerned from FNA smears. However, the introduction of immunocytochemistry led to new classification systems which put much less emphasis on growth patterns and more on immunologic characteristics. In 1988, Tani and coworkers and Ortel and Ortel described the application of immunocytochemistry in the cytologic diagnosis of lymphoma on FNA material. It now seemed possible to conclusively diagnose a majority of lymphomas, which, together with the excellent clinical performance of FNA sampling, should lead to the spread of the technique. Other ancillary techniques such as FISH and PCR have also been applied successfully to FNA material.

This manual has been divided into two chapters which describe the technical and methodological aspects of lymphoma diagnosis, and seven chapters which focus on the cytologic features of neoplastic and reactive lymphoid lesions. We have followed the most recent (2001) WHO lymphoma classification when describing the various lymphoma subtypes. In addition, a separate chapter has been devoted to lymphoma look-alike lesions. Key cytologic and immunologic features are listed to facilitate a conclusive diagnosis of the different lesions.

It is our strong hope that this book will be in the best interest of the patients and will be of help and support to cytopathologists in their diagnostic work with patients with lymphadenopathy of reactive or neoplastic background.

Edneia Tani, Stockholm
Lambert Skoog, Stockholm

Chapter 1

Historical Aspects

Two marine officers, Greig and Gray [1], are recognized as the first to use needle biopsy of lymph nodes. In 1904, they reported that motile trypanosomes could be observed in smears from biopsied nodes. For many years node biopsy was considered a valuable means of demonstrating bubonic plague, trypanosomes and spirochetes. Thus, the technique was only used to identify microorganisms and not to evaluate the cellular components in lymph node disorders.

The first report on lymph node puncture to give a cytomorphologic diagnosis of malignant lymphoma, lymphoblastoma, was published in 1914 by Ward [2]. An attempt to systematically describe cytologic findings in lymph node aspirates from a variety of diseases was presented by Guthrie [3], who as early as 1921 had used air-dried smears stained with Romanowsky. Six years later, Forkner [4] reported on the cytologic presentation of several lymph node disorders in a paper entitled 'Materials from lymph nodes of man'. From then on several papers and monographs were published but the procedure was only slowly accepted by the medical community. In 1952, Morrison et al. [5] reported a large series of lymph node punctures, which included the sensitivity and specificity of the technique. It is puzzling that such an important study had so little impact on the clinical management of patients with lymph node disorders.

In the 1950s and 1960s the development of lymph node cytology was to a large extent the work of clinicians, in particular, those with an interest in hematology. Among them were Pavlowsky, Lopes Cardozo, Abramov, Söderström, and Franzén who all made invaluable contributions [6–10]. However, the clinical background of these pioneers may have been one reason for the slow acceptance of the technique: the pathologists were often unfamiliar with the interpretation of air-dried cells stained with the Romanowsky technique, and also feared that open biopsies could be replaced by fine-needle aspirates. As a consequence, the method was not adopted at most centers for tumor diagnosis in the 1960s.

Several monographs and atlases were however published in the 1960s and 1970s which documented the diagnostic accuracy and wide applicability of fine-needle aspiration cytology. It is of interest to note that even among the enthusiasts and experts in FNA cytology, there seemed to be a discrepancy in the concept of the accuracy of lymphoma diagnosis using cytomorphology alone. Based on a rather limited study, Zajicek [11] concluded that 'about 20% of cases of well-differentiated lymphocytic lymphoma cannot at present be recognized in smears of aspirates'. However, in poorly differentiated (high-grade) lymphoma, he believed that a reliable diagnosis could be made by an experienced examiner.

A somewhat more optimistic but at the same time cautious standpoint was presented by Koss et al. [12] in their textbook in which they state that the question 'Is it or is it not a malignant lymphoma? Can be answered on an aspirate of untreated lesions in most cases'. In fact, the authors believe that 'a precise identification of subtypes of malignant lymphoma can be made by observers with an adequate experience'.

The most optimistic view was expressed by Linsk and Franzén [13] who stated that 'There is no question that the diagnosis can be made with ease by FNA'. Although it may not be all that easy to diagnose lymphomas, one is inclined to believe that it can be made by an experienced examiner after reading the excellent results presented by Lopes Cardozo [14] who accurately diagnosed 1,023 lymphomas on cytology. Moreover, the 'Atlas of clinical cytology' by Lopes Cardozo contains an overwhelming series of beautiful color illustrations of various lymphomas which should make most morphologists interested in lymphoma cytology and accept it as a potentially valuable adjunct to histopathology [15].

The application of immunocytochemistry on lymph node aspirates led to an increased interest in utilizing FNA material for lymphoma diagnosis [16–18]. Simultaneously, it was also shown that immunologic phenotyping of lymphoid cells together with their proliferative characteristics in body cavity effusions enhanced the diagnostic accuracy [19]. With the use of immunocytochemistry, it now became possible to conclusively diagnose lymphoma with an accuracy comparable to that of histopathology. Several studies were published over the following years which confirmed that a cytological diagnosis corroborated by an immunological characterization of the lymphoma cells had a diagnostic accuracy which sometimes not only matched that of histopathology but also surpassed it [20–25].

Subtyping of non-Hodgkin's lymphoma, however, was problematic since the classifications used at this time included growth pattern, i.e. follicular or diffuse, which obviously could not be evaluated on smears.

The situation in the late 1990s has changed dramatically, as the new European American consensus classification (Revised European American classification (REAL) was accepted and replaced all other classifications [26]. This classification is based on clinical, cytologic, immunophenotypic and genetic features and places less emphasis on architectural features. Thus, only follicle center lymphomas are classified with regard to a follicular or diffuse growth pattern. The recognition of pattern is, however, of relative importance in grading but not in diagnosis with one exception, the centroblastic lymphoma. The diffuse subtype is recognized as a variant of diffuse large B cell lymphoma while the follicular variant belongs to the follicle centre lymphoma grade III category. The WHO classification published in 2001 is based on the REAL classification and thus likewise does not place much importance on architectural features [27]. It therefore seems logical that FNA biopsy material, which is an excellent source for cytomorphology, immunology and cytogenetics, could be used not only for diagnosis but also for subtyping of non-Hodgkin lymphoma. This has indeed been confirmed by several studies which all show a high diagnostic accuracy of FNA cytology [28–34].

General Aspects

The cytologic interpretation of smears from lymph node aspirates differs in several respects from that of other organs. Thus, the diagnosis of most solid neoplasms is based on the atypia shown by the tumor cells as compared to their normal counterpart. In contrast, low-grade as well as some high-grade variants of non-Hodgkin lymphomas show little or no cellular atypia and the tumor cells cannot be differentiated from their benign counterparts with certainty. Instead, the cytologic diagnosis is based on the overrepresentation of one or several cell types in the smear. Obviously, such an evaluation can only be made if the spectrum of variation of reactive lymph nodes is fully known. However, even the most experienced cytopathologist cannot reliably diagnose and separate some reactive lymphoid populations from variants of low-grade non-Hodgkin lymphoma on routine smears but also requires ancillary techniques.

In some high-grade lymphomas, smears are dominated by blastic cells which may show only mild cellular atypia. Again the lymphoma diagnosis rests on the overrepresentation of the blastic cells as compared to a reactive lesion, but immunophenotyping should always be used for a conclusive diagnosis and subtyping. Not infrequently, however, the smears from high-grade lymphomas show a highly atypical cell population which on routine smears can only be diagnosed as a high-grade malignant tumor NOS. An immunological evaluation is necessary to reveal the origin of these tumor cells.

Finally, some lymphomas are dominated by benign lymphoid cells, granulocytes or histiocytes. Examples are T cell-rich B cell lymphomas, variants of follicular lymphomas, nodular lymphocyte predominant Hodgkin lymphoma and some cases of classical Hodgkin lymphoma. A correct diagnosis of these variants rests on the identification and cytologic evaluation of only a few tumor cells. In such cases, immunocytochemistry will allow a conclusive diagnosis only if a correct antibody panel has been selected on the basis of a tentative cytological diagnosis.

Today it is clear that cytological diagnoses of lymph node disorders should always be corroborated by an immunological evaluation. This approach is mandatory to reach a sufficiently high diagnostic accuracy for FNA cytology to be accepted for the safe clinical management of patients with lymph node disorders.

Aspirates from lymph nodes suspended in buffered saline offer an excellent material for immunological characterization. Routine FNA sampling yields material enough for numerous analyses. In contrast, direct smears should not be used for immunocytochemistry since such material will often have high background staining which can be detrimental to a correct immunological evaluation.

Immunophenotyping can be performed using flow cytometry or immunocytochemistry on cytospin preparations. Flow cytometry is a rapid and accurate technique for immunological characterization of lymphoid cells and is the method of choice in diagnosing most reactive lympadenopathies as well as low-grade lymphomas. However, blastic lymphomas are often fragile and may be difficult to evaluate using flow cytometry. Moreover Hodgkin lymphomas, T cell-rich B cell lymphomas and nonlymphoid tumors cannot be diagnosed using this technique.

Cytospin preparations allow an immunological evaluation of aspirates from both lymphoid and nonlymphoid lesions of various types. In addition, the equipment used for these techniques is available to most cytology laboratories. The preparation of cytospin material and immunological staining is, however, time consuming, which limits the number of cases that can be processed.

FNA of lymph nodes for primary and follow-up diagnosis with immunophenotyping has been performed at the Division of Clinical Cytology, Karolinska Hospital, Stockholm, since 1986 with an average of 400 lymphoma patients (250 of whom are primary cases) accessioned per year. In this work, immunophenotyping has been performed using either flow cytometry or cytospin preparations.

The excellent performance of FNA cytology in conjunction with immunocytochemistry has been described in several articles. A high rate of both detection and subclassification was demonstrated in a prospective study that included surgical biopsy following FNA of lymph nodes [30]. These results are in agreement with those of others [28, 31–34]. Thus, it is obvious that the diagnostic accuracy of FNA cytology in conjunction with immunophenotyping in trained hands is comparable to that of histopathology.

In situ hybridization and in situ amplification techniques are of importance in both diagnosis and subclassification of some lymphomas [27]. Both techniques are readily applicable to cytologic specimens.

References

1 Greig EDW, Gray ACH: Note on lymphatic glands in sleeping sickness. Lancet 1904;1:1570.
2 Ward GR: Bedside Haematology. Saunders, Philadelphia and London, 1914, p 129.
3 Guthrie CG: Gland puncture as a diagnostic measure. Bull Johns Hopkin's Hosp 1921;32:266–269.
4 Forkner CE: Material from lymph nodes of man. Arch Intern Med 1927;40:532.
5 Morrison M, Samwick AA, Rubinstein J, Stitch M, Loewe L: Lymph node aspiration: clinical and hematologic observations in 101 patients. Am J Clin Pathol 1952;22:255–262.
6 Pavlowsky A: La punción ganglionar: su contribución al diagnóstico clinico-quirúrgico de las afecciones ganglionares; thesis, Buenos Aires A. Lopez, Impr., 1934.
7 Lopes Cardozo P: Clinical Cytology. Leyden, Stafleu, 1954.
8 Abramov MG: Klinitcheskaja Zitologia. Moscow, Medigiz, 1962.
9 Södeström N: Fine Needle Aspiration. Biopsy Stockholm, Almgvist & Wiksell, 1966.
10 Zajicek J, Engzell U, Franzén S: Aspiration biopsy of lymph nodes in diagnosis and research; in Ruttiman A (ed): Progress in Lymphology. Stuttgart, Thieme, 1967, pp 202–264.
11 Zajicek J. In Wied GL (ed): Aspiration Biopsy Cytlogy. Part 1. Monogr Clin Cytol. Basel, Karger, 1974, vol 4.
12 Koss LG, Woyke S, Olszewski W: Aspiration Biopsy. Tokyo, Igaku-Shoin Ltd, 1984.
13 Linsk JA, Franzén S: Clinical Aspiration Cytology. Philadelphia, Lipincott, 1983.
14 Lopes Cardozo P: The significance of fine needle aspiration cytology for the diagnosis and treatment of malignant lymphomas. Folia Hematol 1980;107:602.
15 Lopes Cardozo P. In Lopes Cardozo P (ed): Atlas of Clinical Cytology. Amsterdam, Verlag Chemie, 1975.
16 Martin SE, Zhang HZ, Magyarosy E, Jaffe ES, Hsu S, Chu F: Immunologic methods in cytology: definitive diagnosis of non-Hodgkin's lymphoma using immunologic markers for T and B cells. Am J Clin Pathol 1984;80:666–673.
17 Tani EM, Christensson B, Porwit A, Skoog L: Immunocytochemical analysis and cytomorphologic diagnosis on fine-needle aspirates of lymphoproliferative disease. Acta Cytol 1988;32:209–215.
18 Oertel J, Oertel B, Kastner M, Lobeck H, Huhn D: The value of immunocytochemical staining of lymph node aspirates in diagnostic cytology. Br J Haematol 1988;70:307–316.
19 Katz RL, Raval P. Manning JT, McLaughlin P, Barlogie B: A morphologic, immunologic and cytometric approach to the classification of non-Hodgkin's lymphoma in effusions. Diagn Cytopathol 1987;3:91–101.
20 Tani E, Liliemark J, Svedmyr E, Mellstedt H, Biberfeld P, Skoog L: Cytomorphology and immunocytochemistry of fine-needle aspirates from blastic non-Hodgkin's lymphomas. Acta Cytol 1989;33:363–371.
21 Liliemark J, Tani E, Christensson B, Svedmyr E, Skoog L: Fine-needle aspiration cytology and immunocytochemistry of abdominal non-Hodgkin's lymphomas. Leuk Lymphoma 1989;1:65–69.
22 Skoog L, Tani E: The role of fine needle aspiration cytology in the diagnosis of non-Hodgkin's lymphoma. Diagn Oncol 1991;1:12–18.
23 Cartagena N, Katz RL, Hirsch-Ginsberg C, Childs CC, Odonez NG, Cabanillas F: Accuracy of diagnosis of malignant lymphoma by combining fine-needle aspiration cytomorphology with immunocytochemistry and in selected cases. Southern blotting of aspirated cells: a tissue controlled study of 86 patients. Diagn Cytopathol 1992;8:456–464.
24 Dunphy CH, Ramos R: Combining fine-needle aspiration and flow cytometric immunophenotyping in evaluation of nodal and extranodal sites for possible lymphoma: a retrospective review. Diagn Cytopathol 1997;16:200–206.
25 Young NA, Al-Saleem TI, Ehya H, Smith MR: Utilization of fine needle aspiration cytology and flow cytometry in the diagnosis and subclassification of primary and recurrent lymphoma. Cancer (Cancer Cytopathol) 1998;84:252–261.
26 Harris NL, Jaffe ES, Stein H, et al: A revised European-American classification of lymphoid neoplasms: a proposal from the International Study Group. Blood 1994;84:1361–1392.
27 Jaffe ES, Harris NL, Stein H, Vardiman JW (eds): World Health Organization Classification of Tumors. Pathology and Genetics of Tumours of Haematopoetic and Lymphoid Tissues. Lyon, IARC Press, 2001.
28 Young NA, Al-Saleem TI: Diagnosis of lymphoma by fine-needle aspiration cytology using the Revised European-American classification of lymphoid neoplasms. Cancer (Cancer Cytopathol) 1999;87:325–345.
29 Laane E, Tani E, Björklund E, Elmberger G, Everaus H, Skoog L, Porwit-MacDonald A: Flow cytometric immunophenotyping including Bcl-2 detection on fine needle aspirates in the diagnosis of reactive lymphadenopathy and non-Hodgkin's lymphoma. Cytometry [B] 2005;64:34–42.
30 Landgren O, Porwit Mac Donald A, Tani E, Czader M, Grimfors G, Skoog L, Öst Å, Wedelin C, Axdorph U, Svedmyr E, Björkholm M: A prospective comparison of fine-needle aspiration cytology and histopathology in the diagnosis and classification of lymphomas. Hematol J 2004;5:69–76.
31 Young NA, Al-Saleem T: Diagnosis of lymphoma by fine-needle aspiration cytology using the revised European-American classification of lymphoid neoplasms. Cancer 1999;25;87:325–345.

32 Dong HY, Harris NL, Preffer FI, Pitman MB: Fine-needle aspiration biopsy in the diagnosis and classification of primary and recurrent lymphoma: a retrospective analysis of the utility of cytomorphology and flow cytometry. Mod Pathol 2001;14:472–481.

33 Mourad WA, Tulbah A, Shoukri M, Al Dayel F, Akhtar M, Ali MA, Hainau B, Martin J: Primary diagnosis and REAL/WHO classification of non-Hodgkin's lymphoma by fine-needle aspiration: cytomorphologic and immunophenotypic approach. Diagn Cytopathol 2003;28: 191–195.

34 Zeppa P, Picardi M, Marino G, Troncone G, Fulciniti F, Vetrani A, Rotoli B, Palombini L: Fine-needle aspiration biopsy and flow cytometry immunophenotyping of lymphoid and myeloproliferative disorders of the spleen. Cancer 2003;99:118–127.

Historical Aspects

Chapter 2

Techniques

Fine-Needle Aspiration Biopsy and Smear Preparation

The technique of fine-needle aspiration biopsy has been described in detail in several articles as well as previous textbooks [1–4]. The following presentation is therefore condensed and focused on technical details of particular importance in the collection of lymph node aspiration biopsy material.

Aspiration biopsy of lymph nodes or tumorous lesions should be performed with a thin needle, usually 23–27 gauge (0.6–0.4 mm) fitted to a 10-ml syringe in a one hand grip syringe holder (fig. 2.1). The use of a larger needle should be avoided since it often results in an admixture of peripheral blood which may be detrimental both to cytology and to immunological work-up. The procedure is virtually painless if 23–25 gauge needles are used, and local anesthesia is seldom required. However, in children, we use a local anesthetic cream in most cases (fig. 2.2).

A palpable target is fixed by pressing two fingers horizontally towards it which will immobilize the mass (fig. 2.3). The thumb is used to support the syringe facilitating aspiration of small tumors. Large tumors are fixed between the thumb and the index finger (fig. 2.4). In most cases, one or two needle passes with several [5–10] up and down strokes will procure enough cells for several smears as well as a cell suspension for immunophenotyping and molecular biology.

Nonpalpable lesions, e.g. in the abdomen, lung, mediastinum, orbita, sinuses and bone, are biopsied with the aid of ultrasonography, X-ray or CT. Long 0.5–0.6 mm needles with a stylet are required to reach deep-seated lesions.

Local anesthesia is used when the pleura or peritoneum is penetrated. The needling of deep-seated small targets can

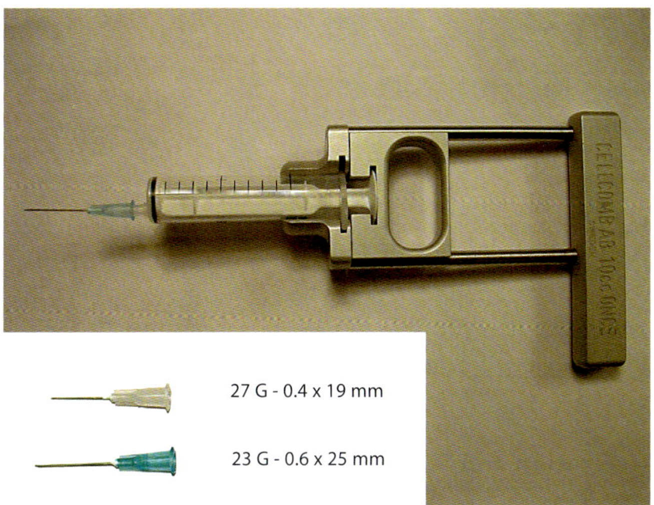

Fig. 2.1. Metal pistol-grip syringe holder and the most commonly used thin needles.

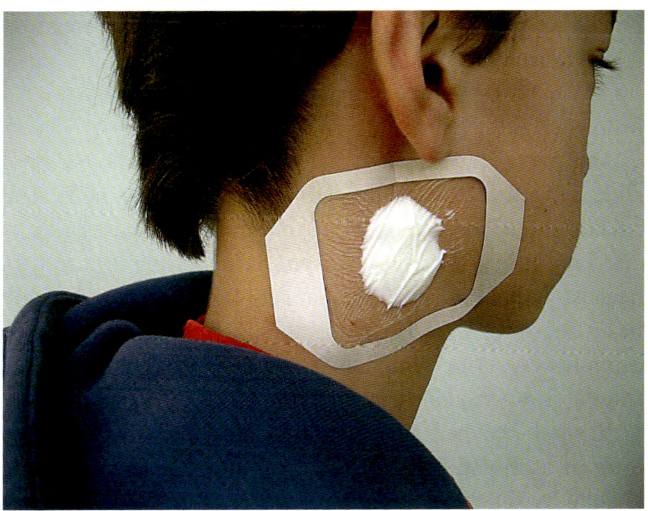

Fig. 2.2. Anesthetic cream applied on the site of puncture.

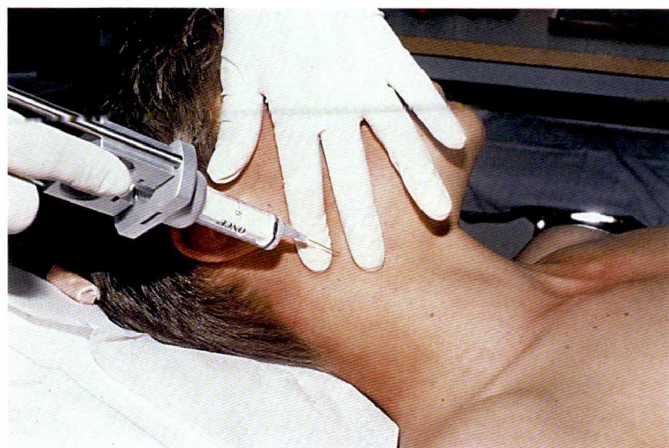

Fig. 2.3. The target is located and fixed by pressing two fingers.

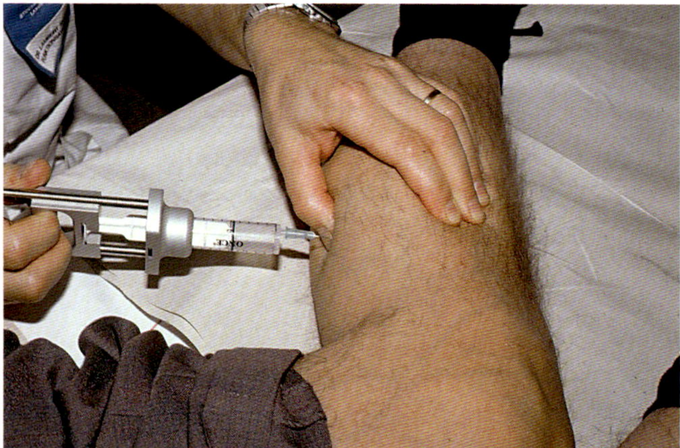

Fig. 2.4. Large palpable targets are fixed between the thumb and the index finger.

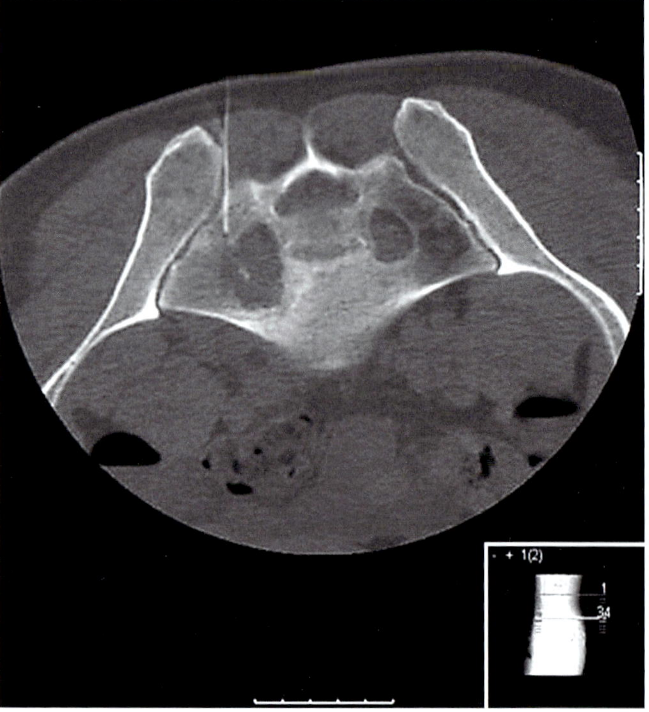

Fig. 2.5. CT-guided FNA biopsy of a nonpalpable lesion in the sacrum with the needle in the correct position. Courtesy of Dr. Veli Söderlund, Clinical Radiology, Karolinska University Hospital.

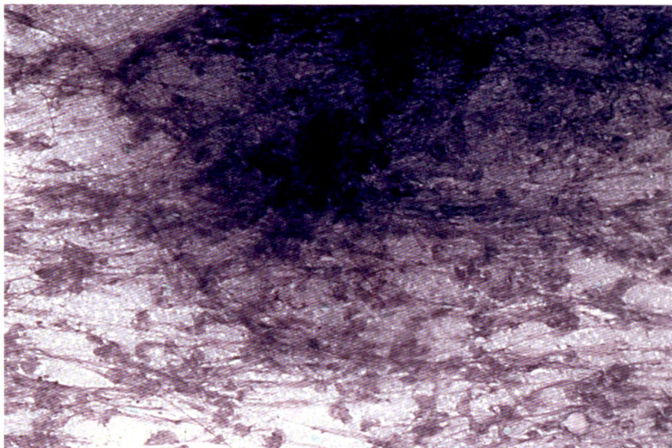

Fig. 2.6. Aspiration smear with fragile crushed cells (MGG, high-power view).

be challenging since long thin needles can be deflected by normal structures. When the needle is in the correct position, the biopsy procedure is similar to that for palpable lesions (fig. 2.5).

One part of the aspirated material is expressed onto a glass slide and smeared carefully with a spreader glass slide. The smears should be even and thin, however care must be exercised not to use too much pressure in preparing thin smears because lymphoid cells are relatively fragile and may easily be crushed (fig. 2.6). The preparation of optimal smears from aspirates of blastic lymphomas, the cells of which are very fragile, is a particularly challenging task.

Several matched smears can be produced from a small drop of aspirated cells using the 'splitting technique'. This is done by touching the drop of aspirated material with the edge of a second glass slide several times. The small droplets are then smeared onto new slides (fig. 2.7). Using this procedure, it is possible to prepare several matched slides from only one aspirate.

Fixation and Staining

Both air-dried and alcohol (ethanol or methanol)-fixed smears should be prepared and stained with May-Grünwald

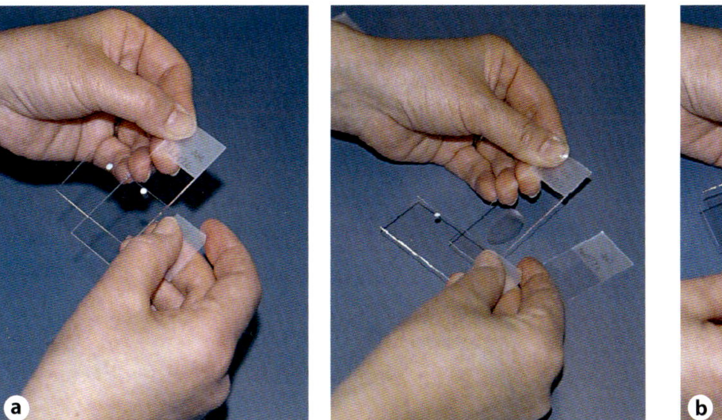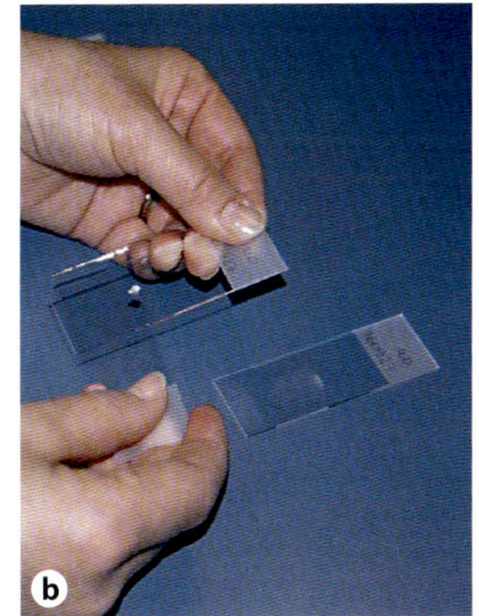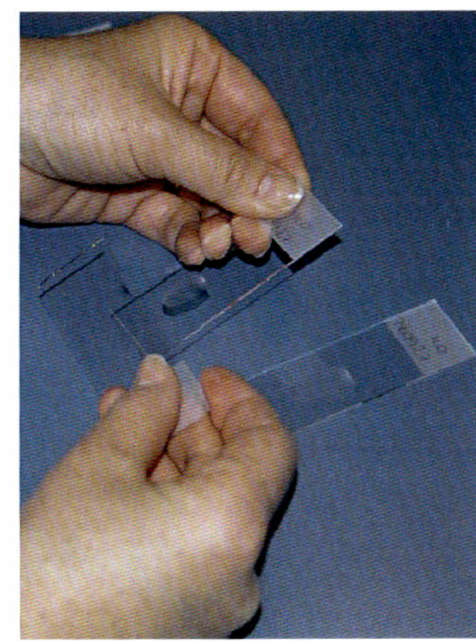

Fig. 2.7. a 'Splitting technique' is done by touching the drop of aspirated material with the edge of the smearing glass (left) and smearing on glass slide (right). **b** The splitted material left on the edge of the smearing glass (left) is smeared on the second glass slide (right).

Giemsa (MGG) stain and Papanicolaou, respectively. An air-dried slide is stained with a 'quick' MGG stain for immediate assessment of cellularity and cell type. The quick stain takes approximately 1.5 min. The smear is stained in May-Grünwald for 45 s followed by 30 s staining in concentrated Giemsa (1:1 dilution with water). Alcohol-fixed smears can also be used for special stains for mycobacteria or fungi. Air-dried smears are well suited for immunocytochemical detection of nuclear proteins such as TdT, cyclin D1, Alk-1, TTF-1, CDX-2, hormone receptors and proliferation marker (MIB-1) after fixation in buffered formalin [5]. Proliferation markers are assessed on smears from all lymphomas as well as other tumors. In addition, air-dried smears can be used for techniques such as FISH although cytospin material generally offers a better source for such analyses.

Fluid Preparation

The pleural and/or peritoneal serous cavities may be involved in patients with lymphoma. Such effusions often contain clotted material which should be removed before the fluid is carefully mixed to produce a homogenous preparation. After the cells have been sedimented at 2,000 g for 10 min, the supernatant is discarded. One part of the sediment is spread on slides, air dried or wet fixed and stained by MGG and PAP, respectively. The remaining material is suspended in phosphate-buffered saline (PBS) and cellularity of the suspension is checked in a Bürker chamber. The number of cells should be adjusted to $1–2 \times 10^6$ cells/ml and the resulting suspension used for cytospin preparation and flow cytometry.

Cytospin Preparation

After using one part of the aspirate to make smears for cytologic diagnosis and for the assessment of cell proliferation, the remaining portion is suspended in 1.5 ml of PBS for cytospin preparation or flow cytometry [6]. This is accomplished by gently aspirating the PBS from the tube through the needle into the syringe. The needle is then disconnected from the syringe and the suspension is then slowly ejected into the tube. The yield of a routine aspirate from an enlarged lymph node may vary between 1 and 10 million cells. This suspension can be analyzed by flow cytometry without adjustment of cellularity (see chap. 3). However, for cytospin preparations, the number of suspended cells should be calculated and the concentration adjusted to $1–2 \times 10^6$ cells/ml before making the cytospin slides. Cell-rich suspensions can be diluted to optimal concentration by adding PBS solution. If the cell concentration is low, a new FNA biopsy is usually performed. If the cell yield still is too low, the cells can be concentrated by centrifugation at 700 rpm for 3–5 min. The resulting pellet is then gently resuspended in a reduced volume of PBS solution and 50–90 µl of the resulting suspension with adjusted cell concentration are used for each cytospin slide.

In most cases, 4 slides with 3 wells are prepared (fig. 2.8). Cells not used for cytospin slides are pelleted and stored frozen for further investigations such as molecular genetics.

One cytospin should be prepared on a regular slide and stained with MGG and compared with the smears to monitor recovery of all cell components (fig. 2.8).

Occasionally, the suspension contains a rich admixture of red blood cells which may interfere with the immunologic

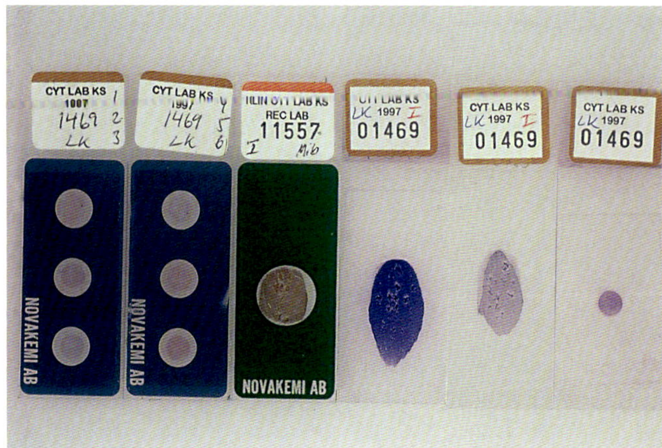
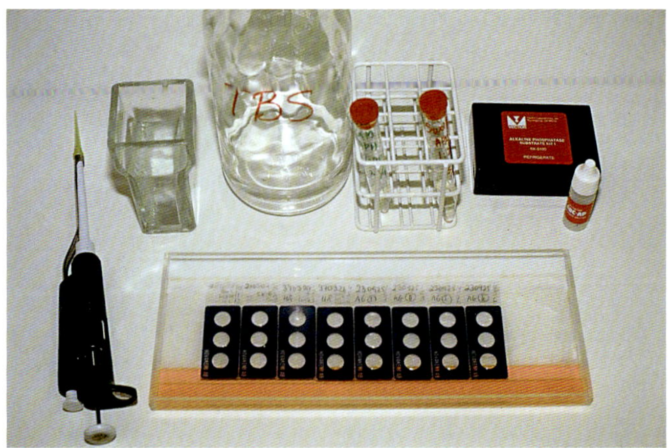

Fig. 2.8. Set of cytological preparation: smears stained with MGG, Papanicolaou and cytospin preparations stained with MGG and several immunostainings.

Fig. 2.9. Immunostaining with alkaline phosphatase technique.

staining. In this case, it is possible to purify the lymphoid cells by density gradient centrifugation in Ficoll-Hypaque® and then use them for cytospin preparations. However, flow cytometry is less sensitive to contaminating blood and is the technique of preference for this type of material.

Storage

Air-dried cytospin preparations can be stored at room temperature for at least 1 week without having a detrimental effect on the immunological staining. Preferably, the cytospins should be stored at −20°C in a plastic box. Under these conditions, lymphoid cells retain their immunological and morphological characteristics for at least several months. For a longer period of storage, −70°C is recommended. Slides which have been stored frozen must be kept in their closed box until fully thawed. Air moisture may otherwise condense on the slides and this will result in poor cell preservation.

Immunostaining

Both immuno-alkaline phosphatase and immuno-peroxidase methods are suitable for cytospin preparations. The high sensitivity and distinct red staining produced with alkaline phosphatase when counterstained with the blue of the hematoxylin stain has made it our procedure of choice [6].

Alkaline phosphatase immunostaining is performed in three steps. Immediately before staining the cells are fixed in acetone (−20°C) for 10 min, air dried and rinsed in Tris-buffered (pH 7.4) saline (TBS) for 5 min. The preparations are incubated with monoclonal antibody in a moist chamber at room temperature for 30 min, followed by rinsing in TBS for 10 min. Alkaline phosphatase-conjugated rabbit anti-mouse Ig is applied for 30 min followed by rinsing. Alkaline phosphatase conjugated swine antiserum to rabbit Ig is then applied for 30 min (fig. 2.9). After rinsing and incubation in alkaline phosphatase developing solution (Vectastain Kit I, Vector Laboratories) for 15–30 min, the slides are washed in water for 5 min and counterstained with Harris hematoxylin. Glycerol gelatin is used as mounting medium.

The selection of the monoclonal antibodies is based on the primary cytomorphologic evaluation and differential diagnoses. In most cases of reactive lymphadenitis and non-Hodgkin lymphoma, a mini-panel of markers is used: anti-kappa, anti-lambda, CD3, CD5, CD10, CD20. A kappa:lambda ratio of 6:1 or a lamba:kappa ratio of 3:1 is considered sufficient to prove monoclonality. Depending on the cytomorphology, monoclonal antibodies are selected from a panel of anti-CD4, CD7, CD8, CD15, CD19, CD23, CD30, CD43, CD45, Bcl-2, pan CK, CK7, CK20, EMA, CEA, HMB45, vimentin, desmin, CD99, NB84, HBME-1, SM actin, chromogranin A, uroplakin and polyclonal antibodies such as S100, PSA, PSAP, thyroglobulin, synaptophysin and calcitonin.

Cell Proliferation

The fraction of cell proliferation is routinely analyzed on an air-dried smear which has been fixed within 4 h in buffered (pH 7.4) formalin for 15 min followed by rinsing in PBS and immersion in ice-cold methanol and acetone for 4 and 1 min, respectively. After rinsing, the slides are incubated with the primary antibody (MIB-1) for 30 min and rinsed in

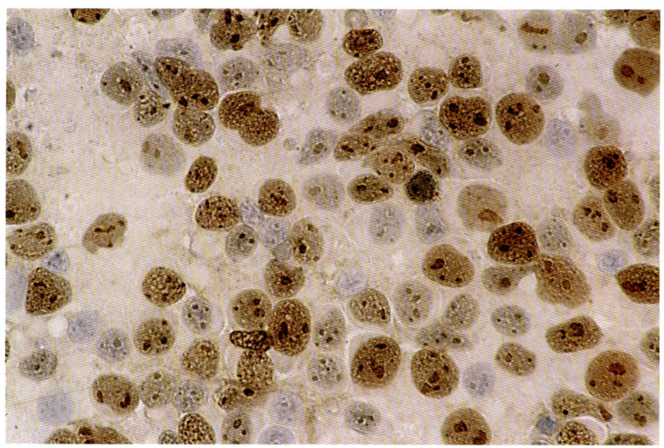

Fig. 2.10. MIB-1 staining of proliferating cells is shown as brown nuclear staining (immunoperoxidase, high-power view).

PBS. The next steps are incubation with the secondary antibody followed by the avidin-biotin-peroxidase (ABC) complex and diamino-benzidine (DAB) The slides are rinsed in PBS between each step.

The evaluation of proliferation by MIB-1 is based on the percentage of positive tumor cells with nuclear staining. If there is a rich admixture of non-neoplastic cells, the rate of proliferation should be corrected accordingly. Two hundred cells are counted and even faint staining is considered positive (fig 2.10). The rate of cell proliferation has been shown to vary both between and within the various subtypes of lymphoma [5, 7–9] and is therefore useful when determining potential aggressiveness.

Molecular Techniques

Molecular analyses supplementary to cytomorphology and immunocytochemistry may be required for diagnosis, subtyping or staging in selected cases (table 2.1). In addition, the molecular analyses will provide information about prognosis and treatment [10 16]. In most cases, fine-needle aspirates provide sufficient material for both cytomorphology, immunocytochemistry and molecular analyses such as polymerase chain reaction (PCR), fluorescence in situ hybridization (FISH) or gene expression profiling by DNA microarray.

Table 2.1. Chromosomal changes in lymphomas

Lymphoma	Cytogenetics
B cell tumors	
Small cell lymphocytic	trisomy 12
Mantle cell	t(11;14)
Marginal zone	trisomy 3, t (11;18)
Follicular	t(14;18)
Burkitt/Burkitt like	t(8;14), t (2;8) or t (8;22)
T cell tumors	
Anaplastic large cell	t(2;5)

It should be stressed that these techniques although relatively easy to set up, need to be meticulously standardized to provide reliable results. In addition, it is important that the results should be integrated with cytologic and immunologic findings.

The PCR technique allows amplification of nucleic acid sequences and can be used to detect monoclonal rearrangements of the IgH or T cell receptor genes [13]. The PCR technique is sensitive and can be used even if the amount of cells is limited. A single FNA sample often contains sufficient material for both cytology and for a cell suspension to be used for immunocytochemistry and PCR. Approximately half the cell suspension can be used to make a cell pellet which is either prepared immediately for PCR or stored frozen for later use.

FISH uses specific probes to detect numerical and structural chromosomal abnormalities in interphase nuclei of tumor cells. This technique is presently used to identify the t(2; 5) in anaplastic large cell lymphoma of the Ki-1 type, t(11; 14) in the mantle cell lymphoma, t(14; 18) in follicle center cell lymphoma, and t (2; 8), t(8; 14) and t(8; 22) in Burkitt lymphoma (table 1). Cytospin material offers an almost ideal cell preparation for FISH analysis.

Gene expression profiling using mRNA hybridization to gene chips will allow a simultaneous analysis of the expression of many genes in neoplastic cells. Results from such studies are likely to allow a more precise subtyping as well as predicting the response to chemotherapy and overall survival. FNA biopsy material has been used successfully to study the gene expression in non-Hodgkin lymphomas [16–18].

References

1 Linsk JA, Franzén S: Introduction; in Linsk JA, Franzéen S (eds): Clinical Aspiration Cytology, ed 2. Philadelphia, Lippincott, 1989.

2 Stanley M, Löwhagen T: Fine Needle Aspiration of Palpable Masses. Boston, Butterworth-Heineman, 1993, pp 1–58.

3 Vielh P: The techniques of FNA cytology; in Orell S, Sterrett G, Walters M, Whitaker D (eds): Fine Needle Aspiration Cytology, ed 3. London, Churchill Livingstone, 1999, pp 9–17.

4 Ljung BM: Techniques of fine needle aspiration, smear preparation and principles of interpretation; in Koss G, Melamed MR (eds): Koss' Diagnostic Cytology and Its Histopathologic Bases, ed 5. Philadelphia, Lippincott, Williams & Wilkins, 2006, pp 1056–1581.

5 Schmitt F, Tani E, Tribukait B, Skoog L: Assessment of cell proliferation by Ki-67 staining and flow cytometry in fine needle aspirates (FNAs) of reactive lymphadenitis and non-Hodgkin's lymphomas. Cytopathology 1999; 10:87–96.

6 Tani E M, Christensson B, Porwit A, Skoog L: Immunocytochemical analysis and cytomorphologic diagnosis on fine-needle aspirates of lymphoproliferative disease. Acta Cytol 1988; 32:209–215.

7 Lorand-Metze I, Pereira FG, Costa FP, Metze K: Proliferation in non-Hodgkin's lymphomas and its prognostic value related to staging parameters. Cell Oncol 2004;26:63–71.

8 Sun W, Caraway NP, Zhang HZ, Khanna A, Payne LG, Katz RL: Grading follicular lymphoma on fine needle aspiration specimens: comparison with proliferative index by DNA image analysis and Ki-67 labeling index. Acta Cytol 2004;48:119–126.

9 Katz RL, Wojcik EM, el-Naggar AK et al: Proliferation markers in non-Hodgkin's lymphoma: a comparative study between cytophotometric quantitation of Ki-67 and flow cytometric proliferation index on fine needle aspirates. Anal Quant Cytol Histol 1993; 15:179–186.

10 Gong Y, Caraway N, Gu J, Zaidi T, Fernandez R, Sun X, Huh YO, Katz RL: Evaluation of interphase fluorescence in situ hybridization for the t(14;18)(q32;q21) translocation in the diagnosis of follicular lymphoma on fine-needle aspirates: a comparison with flow cytometry immunophenotyping. Cancer 2003;25;99:385–393.

11 Bentz JS, Rowe LR, Anderson SR, Gupta PK, McGrath CM: Rapid detection of the t(11;14) translocation in mantle cell lymphoma by interphase fluorescence in situ hybridization on archival cytopathologic material. Cancer 2004; 25;102:124–131.

12 Lee LH, Cioc A, Nuovo GJ: Determination of light chain restriction in fine-needle aspiration-type preparations of B-cell lymphomas by mRNA in situ hybridization. Appl Immunohistochem Mol Morphol 2004;12: 252–258.

13 Safley AM, Buckley PJ, Creager AJ, Dash RC, Dodd LG, Goodman BK, Jones CK, Lagoo AS, Stenzel TT, Wang W, Xie B, Gong JZ: The value of fluorescence in situ hybridization and polymerase chain reaction in the diagnosis of B-cell non-Hodgkin lymphoma by fine-needle aspiration. Arch Pathol Lab Med 2004;128: 1395–1403.

14 Caraway NP, Gu J, Lin P, Romaguera JE, Glassman A, Katz R: The utility of interphase fluorescence in situ hybridization for the detection of the translocation t(11;14) (q13;q32) in the diagnosis of mantle cell lymphoma on fine-needle aspiration specimens. Cancer 2005;25;105:110–118.

15 Kishimoto K, Kitamura T, Fujita K, Tate G, Mitsuya T: Cytologic differential diagnosis of follicular lymphoma grades 1 and 2 from reactive follicular hyperplasia: cytologic features of fine-needle aspiration smears with Pap stain and fluorescence in situ hybridization analysis to detect t(14;18)(q32;q21) chromosomal translocation. Diagn Cytopathol 2006;34: 11–17.

16 Rosenwald A, Wright G, Chan WC, et al: The use of molecular profiling to predict survival after chemotherapy for diffuse large-B-cell lymphoma. N Engl J Med 2002;20;346: 1937–1947.

17 Shipp MA, Ross KN, Tamayo P, et al: Diffuse large B-cell lymphoma outcome prediction by gene-expression profiling and supervised machine learning. Nat Med 2002;8:68–74.

18 Goy A, Stewart J, Barkoh BA, Remache YK, Katz R, Sneige N, Gilles F: The feasibility of gene expression profiling generated in fine-needle aspiration specimens from patients with follicular lymphoma and diffuse large-B-cell lymphoma. Cancer 2006;108:10–20.

....

Chapter 3

Flow Cytometry in Fine-Needle Aspiration Diagnosis of Lymphomas

Immunophenotyping is essential in fine-needle aspiration (FNA) diagnosis of lymphoma. It can easily be accomplished via multiparameter flow cytometry (FC), which is a rapid and sensitive method to evaluate lymphoid markers. FC appears to be especially useful in FNA specimens from lymphoid tissues and other infiltrates suspected of lymphoma, from which single-cell suspensions can be easily obtained. It is also often applied in fluid samples where cells are naturally suspended (blood, bone marrow, cerebrospinal fluid, ascites, pleural fluid) [1, 2]. Cells in suspension are stained with antibodies conjugated with fluorescent markers that emit light at different wavelengths, thus allowing detection of multiple marker expression in each cell. At the moment four-color FC is a standard method in immunophenotyping of lymphomas, but polychromatic FC where up to 17 fluorochromes can be employed is developing rapidly [3]. Evaluation of scattering of light (forward scatter – FSC, and side scatter – SSC) properties allows elimination of dead and apoptotic cells as well as granulocytes. Combination of scatter characteristics and lineage-associated markers (CD19 and/or CD7 or CD3) makes it possible to investigate subpopulations of B and T cells, and to achieve subclassifications of lymphomas.

FC requires only a small sample, gives quantitative results and can detect small abnormal cell populations in a reactive background. Moreover, if necessary, FC results can be obtained within a couple of hours from the time of biopsy. The usual turnaround time is 1 working day.

Several studies have evaluated FC immunophenotyping in FNA material showing a high detection rate of NHL (table 3.1) [4–20]. All these studies showed good agreement with the histopathological diagnoses on surgical biopsies. The proportion of samples correctly diagnosed and classified by FC has been increasing from 70–80% in the early studies and in cases of high-grade or T cell lymphomas to almost 100% in the latest publications.

Methodological Considerations

Sample Preparation

The four-color FC method applied in our department has been previously described in detail [20]. A stain and then lyse/wash technique is used. The optimal number of cells per tube is approximately 1×10^6, which may be difficult to achieve in everyday practice. At minimum, approximately 50×10^3 cells can be stained to acquire and analyze $5–10 \times 10^3$ 'events'.

Antibody Panel

It is evident from the literature that the sensitivity and specificity of lymphoma detection increase with the number of fluorochromes applied. Four four-color monoclonal antibodies extensively tested by us are presented in table 3.2 and illustrated in figure 3.1. Recently, we have replaced this panel with a one four-color/seven MAB combination (table 3.3; fig. 3.2). This panel is very efficient in samples with only few cells and quickly provides information on the presence of a monoclonal B cell population in the sample. When a population suspect for lymphoma is present, an additional tube(s) (usually Bcl-2 FITC/CD10PE/CD20 PerCP/ CD5 APC) is analyzed to further determine the immunophenotype of monoclonal B cells.

In the Bcl-2 expression analysis, the staining for surface markers is followed by a fixation and permeabilization with Intrastain (Dako), according to the manufacturer's recommendation [20]. We found that inclusion of Bcl-2 into the FC panel was useful, since, in most samples, malignant B cells had higher levels of Bcl-2 expression than reactive B cells. In cases of FL or high-grade NHL where malignant B cells often showed overexpression of Bcl-2, it was possible to detect a malignant population in a substantial reactive background (fig. 3.1, row 4, right plot).

Table 3.1. Diagnostic accuracy in reported studies on FC application in immunophenotyping of FNA specimens

Reference, year	Number of NHL samples	Number of reactive samples	Number of fluorochromes	Diagnostic sensitivity of FC, %	WHO/REAL subclassification accuracy, %
Robins et al. [4], 1994	71	0	2	92	NA
Dunphy and Ramos [5], 1997	60	8	2	80	NA
Young et al. [6], 1998	50		2	80	NA
Henrique et al. [7], 1999	61	11	2	60/88[1]	78
Liu et al. [8], 1999	22[2]	0	3	100	NA
Ravinsky et al. [9], 1999	41	11	2	85.5	88
Simsir et al. [30], 1999	70	6	3	89	88
Al Shangeety and Mourad [10], 2000	20[3]	0	2	80	NA
Meda et al. [11], 2000	158	81	2	95	100[4]
Nicol et al. [12], 2000	156	71	3	93	94
Cannon and Richardson [13], 2001	49[5]	20	NA	86	86
Dong et al. [14], 2001	105	0	4	74	77
Liu et al. [15], 2001	117	27	3	98	77
Yao et al. [16], 2001	21[3]	0	2	72	NA
Mourad et al. [17], 2003	53	0	4	100	80
Sigstad et al. [18], 2004	17	41	2–4	NA	59%[6]
Zeppa et al. [19], 2004	147	135	2 or 3	93	63
Laane et al. [20], 2005	239	172	4	78/95[1]	89.5

NA = Not available.
[1] High-grade/low-grade B-NHL.
[2] Intra-abdominal localization.
[3] T cell NHL only.
[4] B cell NHL only.
[5] Head and neck, private practice, commercial FC laboratory.
[6] Referred cases sent by mail only.

Table 3.2. Four-tube four-color panel of monoclonal antibodies for FNA lymphoma diagnostics*

Tube	FITC	PE	PerCP alt. PE-Cy5	APC
1	CD23	CD10	CD20	CD19
2	lambda	kappa	CD19	CD5
3	CD4	CD7	CD8	CD3
4	Bcl-2	CD10	CD19	CD3

* According to Laane et al. [20].
FITC = Fluorescein isothiocyanate; PE = R-phycoerythrin; PerCP = peridinin chlorophyll protein; PE-Cy5 = tandem conjugate system which combines R-phycoerythrin and a cyanine dye; APC = allophycocyanin

Data Analysis
Most FNA aspirates from lymph nodes or other lymphatic tissue contain normal lymphocytes, which serve as a reference for scatter and staining analysis. Small reactive T cells have low FSC and SSC characteristics (fig. 3.1, row 2, left plot). Both reactive germinal center B cells and neoplastic B cells of low-grade lymphomas can be larger in size (fig. 3.1, row 1, middle plot and row 3, left plot). Especially in diffuse large B cell lymphomas, diagnostic information may be obtained by gating on large B cells separately (fig. 3.3).

The most important part of the analysis is assessing clonality of B cells (fig. 3.1, 3.2). The light chain expression should be assessed in CD19 versus SSC gate, corrected for adequate FSC (fig. 3.1, row 3, left and middle plot, fig. 3.2, upper right and lower left plot). In our study, the median kappa/lambda ratio in reactive lymphatic tissue was 1.6 (range 0.4–4.7). In practice, a ratio under 0.6 and above 6.0 is considered suspicious. Additional analyses can be performed looking for clonal B cells in CD10+/CD19+ or CD5+/CD19+ cells or CD19/large cell FSC/SSC gate or for Bcl-2 overexpressing B cells. However, in rare lymph nodes with reactive follicular hyperplasia, light chain restriction may occur within a CD10+ B cell population without overexpression of bcl-2 or t(14,18) [21]. Another aberrant finding commonly encountered in lymphomas is the presence of

Flow Cytometry in Fine-Needle Aspiration
Diagnosis of Lymphomas

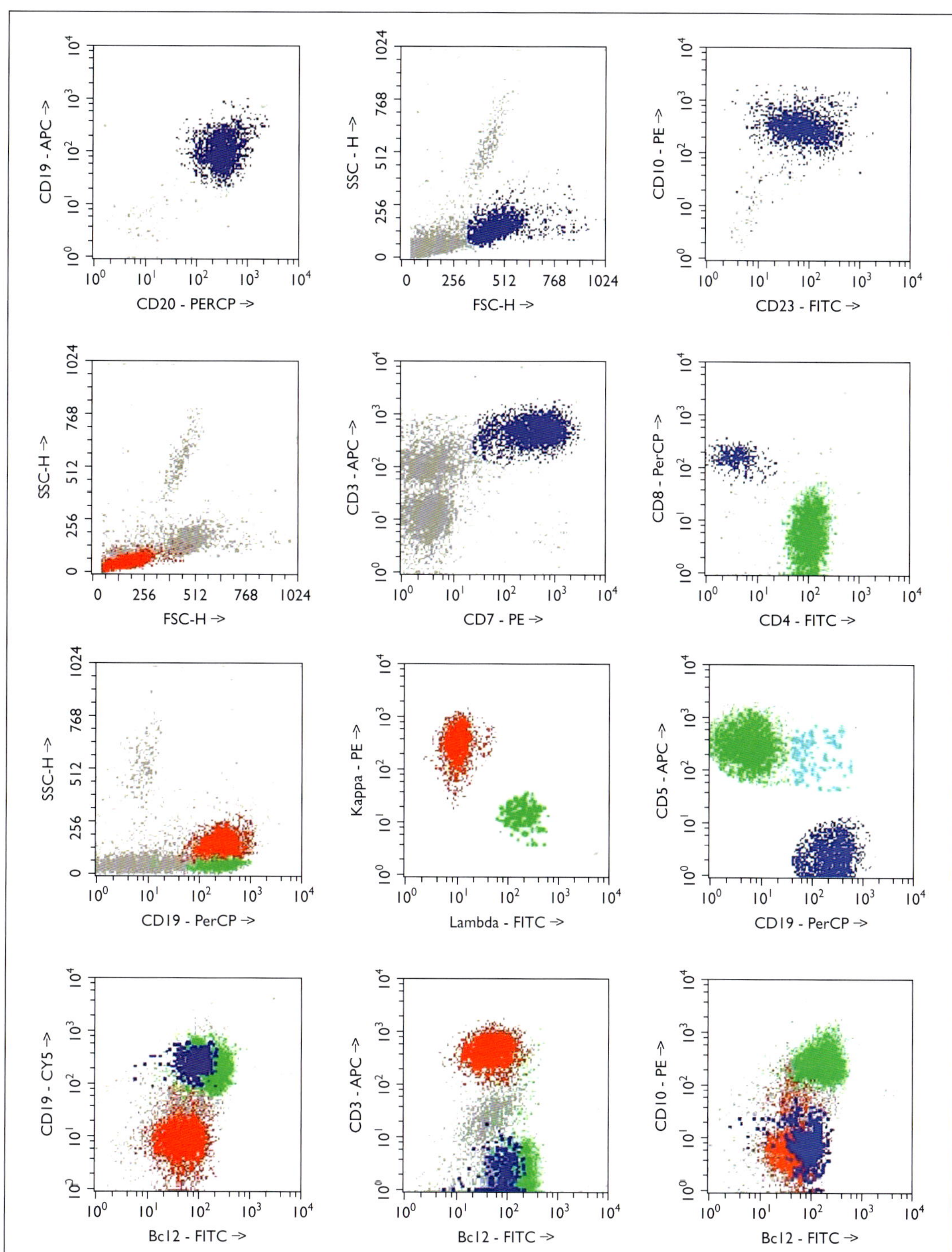

Fig. 3.1. FC diagnostics of lymphomas using a panel of four 4-color MAB combinations listed in table 3.2. Example of analysis of FNΛ from a lymph node involved by a follicular lymphoma. Row 1 shows analysis of the first tube where a large population of CD19/CD20-positive cells (left plot, blue dots) was found. These cells are larger than T lymphocytes (middle plot) and positive for CD10 and CD23 (right plot). Row 2 shows analysis of tube 3 where T cells present in the sample are smaller than B cells (left plot, red dots) and show normal expression of CD3 and CD7 (middle plot, blue dots), and normal CD4/CD8 ratio (right plot: CD4+ red dots, CD8+ green dots). Row 3 shows analysis of tube 2. After CD19/SSC gating (left plot) there is a dominance of kappa+ B cells (red dots), but a population of lambda-+ B cells is also present (green dots). Note that kappa+ have different scatter compared to lambda positive ones (left plot). Only a minimal population of CD5+ B cells is present (mantle zone cells, right plot, cyan dots). Row 4 shows Bcl-2 analysis (tube 4) where CD10+ cells (green dots) have stronger Bcl-2 expression when compared to CD10− B cells (blue dots) and CD3+ T cells (red dots).

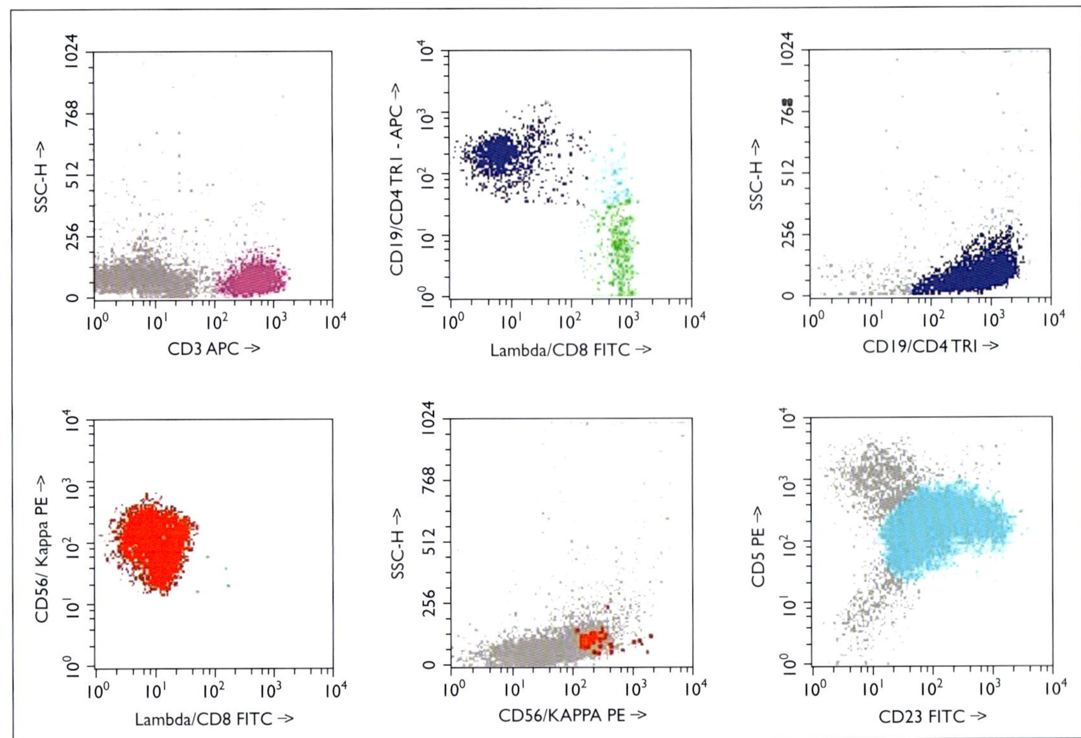

Fig. 3.2. FC diagnostics of lymphomas using panel of a four-color seven-MAB combination listed in table 3.3. Example of analysis of a FNA from a lymph node involved by a B-CLL type lymphocytic lymphoma. Left upper plot shows the first step of analysis – gating of CD3+ T cells (violet dots). Upper middle plot shows rather high CD4/CD8 ratio (CD4+ blue dots, CD8+ green dots) and a presence of a minimal CD4/CD8 double-positive population (cyan dots). After this analysis CD3+ cells are electronically removed and CD19+ cells are gated from the remaining population (right upper plot, blue dots). Light chain analysis within CD19+ population (lower left plot, kappa: red dots, lambda: green dots) shows that B cells were monoclonal for kappa. Lower middle plot shows a few CD56+ cells (red dots) that can be painted after both CD3+ cells and CD19+ B cells are removed. Red-painted CD56+ cells are visualized after all cells are restored. Due to the presence of a monoclonal B cell population, an additional tube has been stained (CD23 FITC/CD5PE/CD19PECy5/ CD10APC) showing that almost all B cells were positive for CD5 and CD23 (right lower plot, cyan dots).

Table 3.3. One-tube four-color panel of seven monoclonal antibodies for FNA lymphoma diagnostics*

Tube	FITC	PE	PE Cy5/PerCP	APC
1	lambda and CD8	kappa and CD56	CD19 and CD4	CD3

*According to Costa et al. [31].

a B cell population lacking surface light chain expression. This can be seen in B precursor leukemia/lymphoma, CLL, DLCB or plasma cell proliferations. In the latter category of cases, additional analysis of cytoplasmic light chain expression may show a clonal B cell population [22].

Evaluation of Bcl-2 expression is helpful in lymphoma cases with partial involvement and presence of reactive germinal centers, which makes evaluation of light chain restriction difficult [20, 23, 24]. In the applied MAB combination (table 3.2) Bcl-2 expression is evaluated simultaneously in B and T cells and, if present, in CD10+ B cells. In this approach, nonmalignant T cells present in the sample serve as internal control for the comparison of the levels of Bcl-2 expression (fig. 3.1, row 4). The presence of CD10+ B cells with high Bcl-2 expression is highly predictive for follicular lymphoma. In contrast, CD10+ B cells in reactive lymphatic tissue show a lower level of Bcl-2 expression than T cells and CD10-negative B cells (fig. 3.4). Increased Bcl-2 expression is also found in most CD10-negative low-grade B cell lymphomas [20]. In DLCB lymphomas, Bcl-2 expression is not as informative since malignant B cells may be Bcl-2-negative [25].

The immunophenotypic criteria for diagnosis of various B cell lymphoma subtypes are summarized in table 3.4 and discussed in detail in the respective chapters. Our FC panel is very useful in detecting low-grade B cell lymphomas (96% of cases diagnosed and classified accurately) [20].

Flow Cytometry in Fine-Needle Aspiration
Diagnosis of Lymphomas

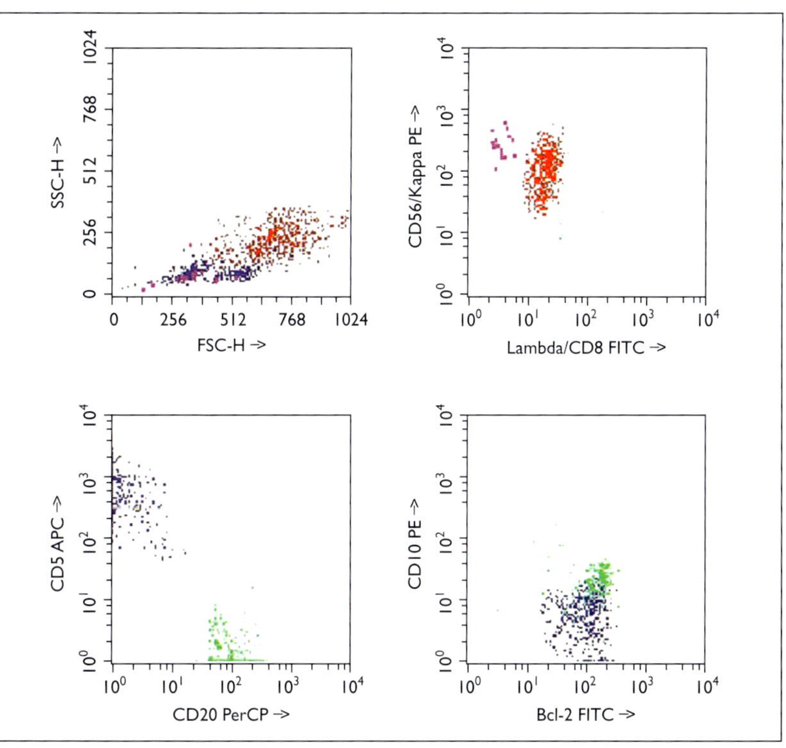

Fig. 3.3. FC immunophenotyping of fine-needle aspirate from a lymph node with diffuse large B cell lymphoma. Four-color FC was used. Upper left plot shows forward scatter/side scatter image of the sample with kappa+ B cells (red dots) being considerably larger in size than CD3+ T lymphocytes (blue dots). Upper right plot shows a dominance of large kappa+ B cells within the B cell population (gating on CD19 = side scatter; red dots – kappa | large cells; – violet dots = kappa+ small cells; green dots = lambda + cells). Lower left plot shows that CD20+ B cells (green dots) were less numerous than T cells (blue dots) (30 and 50%, respectively) and that B cells were negative for CD5. Lower right plot shows that most B cells (green dots) were negative for CD10 and that Bcl-2 expression was similar in B and T cells (blue dots).

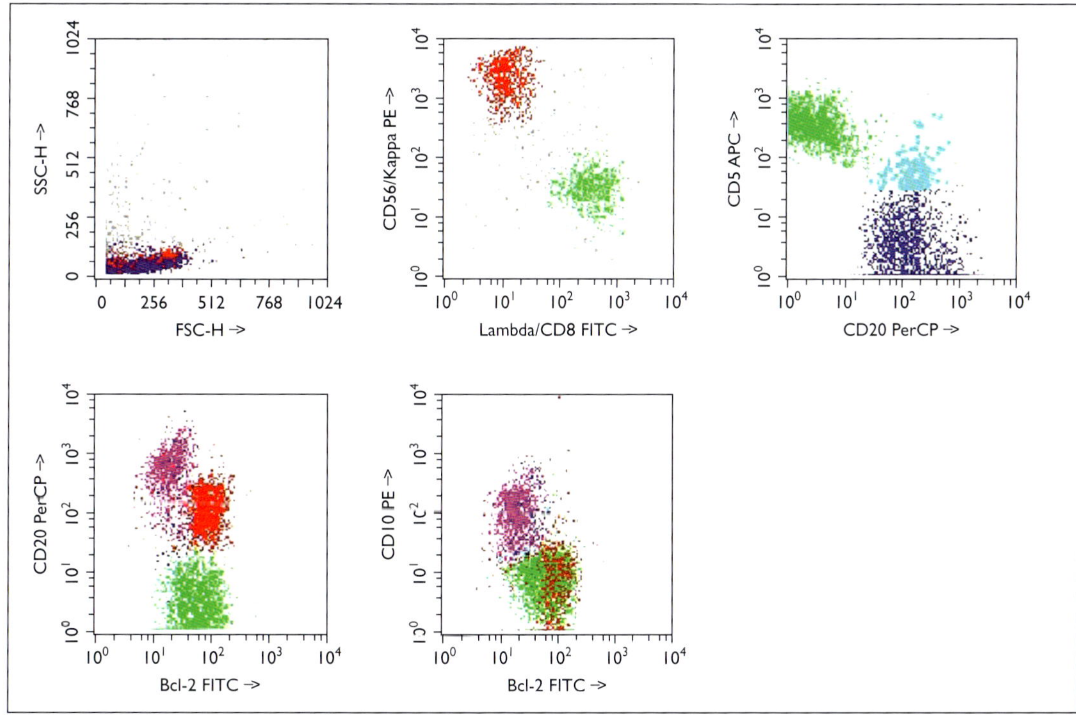

Fig. 3.4. FC immunophenotyping of fine-needle aspirate from a lymph node with a reactive follicular hyperplasia. Four-color FC was used. Upper left plot shows forward scatter/side scatter image of the sample with CD20+ B cells (red dots) being similar in size to CD5+ T lymphocytes (blue dots). Upper middle plot shows that B cells were polyclonal with a presence of kappa+ B cells and lambda+ B cells (gating on CD19 = side scatter; red dots = kappa+ cells; green dots = lambda+ cells). Upper right plot shows a presence of a small CD5+ population of B cells corresponding to normal mantle-zone cells (cyan dots). Lower left plot shows that most CD20+ B cells (red dots) had similar Bcl-2 expression to CD5+ T cells (green dots), but there is a subpopulation of CD20+ cells with higher CD20 expression and lower Bcl-2 (violet dots). These cells correspond to CD10+ germinal center B cells with low Bcl-2 expression as illustrated on the right lower plot.

Table 3.4. Immunophenotypic criteria for the diagnosis and classification of B-cell Non-Hodgkin lymphoma and reactive hyperplasia in FNA*

Diagnosis	CD19	CD5	CD23	CD20	CD10	K/L
FL	+	−	−	+	+	clonal
CLL	+	+	+	+ (weak)	−	clonal
IC/LPL	+	−	−	+	−	clonal
MALT/NMZL	+	−	−	+	−	clonal
MCL	+	+	−	+	−	clonal
HG-NHL	+	−	−/+	+/−	+/−	clonal
RH	+	−	−/+	+/−	−/+	polyclonal

*According to Laane et al. [20].
FL = Follicular lymphoma; CLL = chronic lymphocytic leukemia; IC/LPL = immunocytoma/lymphoplasmocytic lymphoma; MALT/NMZL = extranodal marginal zone B cell lymphoma of mucosa-associated lymphoid tissue type/nodal marginal zone lymphoma; MCL = mantle cell lymphoma; HG-NHL = high-grade B cell non-Hodgkin lymphoma; RH = reactive hyperplasia; K/L = kappa/lambda light chain ratio.

Table 3.5. Aberrant features often found in FNA aspirates from T cell lymphomas

Aberrant feature	Type of T-NHL	References
CD4/CD8 ratio above 15	cutaneous NHL, peripheral T cell	Laane et al. [20]
CD4/CD8 double-negative	T precursor, peripheral T-NHL	Herling et al. [27], Porwit-MacDonald et al. [32]
CD4/CD8 double-positive	T-PLL	Herling et al. [27]
CD4−/CD8+	hepatosplenic gamma/delta, large granular lymphocyte leukemia	Ahmad et al. [33]
CD4+/CD7− phenotype	cutaneous, peripheral T	Herling et al. [27]
TdT+	precursor T	Bardales et al. [34], Porwit-MacDonald et al. [32]
CD3 dim/negative	precursor T, peripheral T	Stetler-Stevenson [2], Porwit-MacDonald et al. [32], Edelman and Meyerson [35]
CD2 dim/negative, CD5 dim/negative	precursor T, peripheral T	Porwit-MacDonald et al. [32], Jamal et al. [36]
CD10+ T-cells	angioimmunoblastic T	Attygalle et al. [28], Lee et al. [37]
CD56+	hepatosplenic gamma/delta and T/NK nasal type	Ahmad et al. [33]
CD57+	large granular lymphocyte leukemia	Ahmad et al. [33]
CD25++	adult T cell leukemia, lymphoma	Dahmoush et al. [38]
CD20+	rare peripheral T cell lymphomas	Yokose et al. [39]
CD26 negative T cells	cutancous NHL	Jones et al. [40]

CD10 negative follicular lymphomas are the only problematic category. Grade III and interfollicular infiltrating cells in other FC may lack CD10 and in these cases the lymphoma subtype maybe misdiagnosed by FC [26]. Approximately 10% of FLs are reported to be CD10−.

T cell lymphomas are usually more difficult to analyze by FC than B cell lymphomas due to their very variable patterns of antigen expression. The most common aberrant findings are summarized in table 3.5. Most often, T cell lymphomas show imbalance in CD4/CD8 ratio and/or aberrant expression

Flow Cytometry in Fine-Needle Aspiration
Diagnosis of Lymphomas

of one or more 'pan-T cell' markers as CD2, CD3, CD5 or CD7 [27]. Aberrant expression of CD10 is found in T cells in angioimmunoblastic T cell NHL [28]. It has to be noted that increased CD4/CD8 ratios, sometimes with an activated pattern (CD25+), and very low frequency of polyclonal B cells can be found in FNA samples from Hodgkin lymphomas which could lead to a misdiagnosis of T cell lymphoma [2].

Recently, a direct analysis of T cell clonality by FC analysis of T cell receptor V-beta chain expression has been made possible [29]. However, even with this approach, some obvious T cell lymphoproliferations were negative for clonality and in some reactive cases dominant T cell populations with polyclonal background were found.

Advantages and Disadvantages of FC

Immunophenotyping by FC has several advantages. FC is rapid, sensitive, gives quantitative results and allows antigens to be assessed simultaneously. Therefore, various subpopulations of lymphocytes can be analyzed separately with high sensitivity. Small abnormal cell populations can be detected in a reactive background. FC allows detection of antigen expression on the cell surface, which is of importance when planning antibody-based therapy such as Rituximab, Campath or Daclizumab, as the antigens (CD20, CD52, CD4 respectively) have to be expressed on the cell surface for the therapy to be effective.

However, it may be difficult to assess which cells in cytologic preparations correspond to different populations detected by FC. Staining for intracellular markers (intracytoplasmic and nuclear) may produce high levels of background and analysis may need a high level of expertise. Inadequate sampling, fibrosis, and necrosis may result in nonrepresentative samples.

The main disadvantage of FC is its unawareness of cytomorphology. The size of cells can only be assessed approximately. Also, if neoplastic cells are fragile as in many high-grade NHL and in Hodgkin lymphoma, they may be destroyed during FC analysis. Grading of follicular lymphoma and detection of transformation to DLCB is possible only by morphology. For that reason close cooperation between cytopathologists and FC laboratory is required.

Comparison between FC and Immunocytochemistry on Cytospins

Three large studies have compared the results of immunocytochemistry (IC) on cytospins and FC [4, 20, 30]. All point out the excellent correlation of obtained results (85–97%). The main advantage of IC over FC is that it requires lower numbers of cells and that staining pattern, intensity of staining and background can be assessed by morphology. Fragile cells that disappear during FC preparation can usually be assessed in cytospins. However, preparation artifacts, necrosis, increased blood contamination and background staining can render an accurate evaluation of cytospin preparation difficult. Also, immunocytochemistry is relatively time consuming (approx. 3 times longer technician time is required). Moreover, routinely it is not possible to evaluate multiple antigen expression and scoring is semiquantitative.

How to Get the Best Results in FC Diagnostics of FNA

Based on our experience, we recommend quick staining of one smear from the FNA sample for immediate evaluation. If small- to medium-sized cells predominate, indicating low-grade lymphoma or a reactive process, FC should be the method of choice for immunophenotyping. When large cells predominate, IC is preferable since FC has a high false-negative rate. Hodgkin lymphoma, anaplastic large-cell lymphoma and some high-grade NHL-like T cell-rich B cell lymphomas cannot be reliably detected by FC. Close cooperation and communication between the cytopathologist and FC laboratory is a prerequisite for a high diagnostic accuracy. It is also of importance that adequate material is saved (frozen cells or cytopsins) for FISH or molecular genetics studies.

References

1 Dunphy CH: Applications of flow cytometry and immunohistochemistry to diagnostic hematopathology. Arch Patohol Lab Med 2004; 128:1004–1022.
2 Stetler-Stevenson M: Flow cytometry in lymphoma diagnosis and prognosis: useful? Best Pract Res Clin Haematol 2003;16:583–597.
3 Perfetto SP, Chattopadhyay PK, Roederer M: Seventeen-colour flow cytometry: unravelling the immune system. Nat Rev Immunol 2004; 4:648–655.
4 Robins DB, et al: Immunotyping of lymphoma by fine-needle aspiration. A comparative study of cytospin preparations and flow cytometry. Am J Clin Pathol 1994;101:569–576.
5 Dunphy CH, Ramos R: Combining fine-needle aspiration and flow cytometric immunophenotyping in evaluation of nodal and extranodal sites for possible lymphoma: a retrospective review. Diagn Cytopathol 1997;16: 200–206.
6 Young NA, et al: Utilization of fine-needle aspiration cytology and flow cytometry in the diagnosis and subclassification of primary and recurrent lymphoma. Cancer 1998;84: 252–261.
7 Henrique RM, et al: Immunophenotyping by flow cytometry of fine needle aspirates in the diagnosis of lymphoproliferative disorders: a retrospective study. J Clin Lab Anal 1999;13: 224–228.

8 Liu K, et al: Fine-needle aspiration with flow cytometric immunophenotyping for primary diagnosis of intra abdominal lymphomas. Diagn Cytopathol 1999;21:98–104.

9 Ravinsky E, et al: Cytodiagnosis of lymphoid proliferations by fine needle aspiration biopsy. Adjunctive value of flow cytometry. Acta Cytol 1999;43:1070–1078.

10 Al, Shanqeety O, Mourad WA: Diagnosis of peripheral T-cell lymphoma by fine-needle aspiration biopsy: a cytomorphologic and immunophenotypic approach. Diagn Cytopathol 2000;23:375–379.

11 Meda BA, et al: Diagnosis and subclassification of primary and recurrent lymphoma. The usefulness and limitations of combined fine-needle aspiration cytomorphology and flow cytometry. Am J Clin Pathol 2000;113:688–699.

12 Nicol TL, et al: The accuracy of combined cytopathologic and flow cytometric analysis of fine-needle aspirates of lymph nodes. Am J Clin Pathol 2000;114:18–28.

13 Cannon CR, Richardson LD: Value of flow cytometry in the evaluation of head and neck fine-needle lymphoid aspirates: a 3-year retrospective review of a community-based practice. Otolaryngol Head Neck Surg 2001;124:544–548.

14 Dong HY, et al: Fine-needle aspiration biopsy in the diagnosis and classification of primary and recurrent lymphoma: a retrospective analysis of the utility of cytomorphology and flow cytometry. Mod Pathol 2001;14:472–481.

15 Liu K, et al: Diagnosis of hematopoietic processes by fine-needle aspiration in conjunction with flow cytometry: A review of 127 cases. Diagn Cytopathol 2001;24:1–10.

16 Yao JL, et al: Fine-needle aspiration biopsy of peripheral T-cell lymphomas. A cytologic and immunophenotypic study of 33 cases. Cancer 2001;93:151–159.

17 Mourad WA, et al: Primary diagnosis and REAL/WHO classification of non-Hodgkin's lymphoma by fine-needle aspiration: cytomorphologic and immunophenotypic approach. Diagn Cytopathol 2003;28:191–195.

18 Sigstad E, et al: The role of flow cytometric immunophenotyping in improving the diagnostic accuracy in referred fine-needle aspiration specimens. Diagn Cytopathol 2004;31:159–163.

19 Zeppa P, et al: Fine-needle cytology and flow cytometry immunophenotyping and subclassification of non-Hodgkin lymphoma: a critical review of 307 cases with technical suggestions. Cancer 2004;102:55–65.

20 Laane E, et al: Flow cytometric immunophenotyping including Bcl-2 detection on fine needle aspirates in the diagnosis of reactive lymphadenopathy and non-Hodgkin's lymphoma. Cytometry [B] 2005;64:34–42.

21 Kussick SJ, et al: Prominent clonal B-cell populations identified by flow cytometry in histologically reactive lymphoid proliferations. Am J Clin Pathol 2004;121:464–472.

22 Ocqueteau M, et al: Immunophenotypic characterization of plasma cells from monoclonal gammopathy of undetermined significance patients. Implications for the differential diagnosis between MGUS and multiple myeloma. Am J Pathol 1998;152:1655–1665.

23 Cornfield DB, et al: Follicular lymphoma can be distinguished from benign follicular hyperplasia by flow cytometry using simultaneous staining of cytoplasmic bcl-2 and cell surface CD20. Am J Clin Pathol 2000;114:258–263.

24 Cook JR, Craig FE, Swerdlow SH: bcl-2 expression by multicolor flow cytometric analysis assists in the diagnosis of follicular lymphoma in lymph node and bone marrow. Am J Clin Pathol 2003;119:145–151.

25 Hermine O, et al: Prognostic significance of bcl-2 protein expression in aggressive non-Hodgkin's lymphoma. Groupe d'Etude des Lymphomes de l'Adulte (GELA). Blood 1996;87:265–272.

26 Eshoa C, et al: Decreased CD10 expression in grade III and in interfollicular infiltrates of follicular lymphomas. Am J Clin Pathol 2001;115:862–867.

27 Herling M, et al: A systematic approach to diagnosis of mature T-cell leukemias reveals heterogeneity among WHO categories. Blood 2004;104:328–335.

28 Attygalle A, et al: Neoplastic T cells in angioimmunoblastic T-cell lymphoma express CD10. Blood 2002;99:627–633.

29 Morice WG, et al: Flow cytometric assessment of TCR-Vbeta expression in the evaluation of peripheral blood involvement by T-cell lymphoproliferative disorders: a comparison with conventional T-cell immunophenotyping and molecular genetic techniques. Am J Clin Pathol 2004;121:373–383.

30 Simsir A, et al: Immunophenotypic analysis of non-Hodgkin's lymphomas in cytologic specimens: a correlative study of immunocytochemical and flow cytometric techniques. Diagn Cytopathol 1999;20:278–284.

31 Costa ES, Arroyo ME, Pedreira CE, García-Marcos MA, Tabernero MD, Almeida J, Orfao A: A new automated flow cytometry data analysis approach for the diagnostic screening of neoplastic B-cell disorders in peripheral blood samples with absolute lymphocytosis. Leukemia 2006;20:1221–1230.

32 Porwit-MacDonald A, et al: BIOMED-1 concerted action report: flow cytometric characterization of CD7+ cell subsets in normal bone marrow as a basis for the diagnosis and follow-up of T cell acute lymphoblastic leukemia (T-ALL). Leukemia 2000;14:816–825.

33 Ahmad E, et al: Flow cytometric immunophenotypic profiles of mature gamma delta T-cell malignancies involving peripheral blood and bone marrow. Cytometry B Clin Cytom 2005;67:6–12.

34 Bardales RH, et al: Detection of terminal deoxynucleotidyl transferase (TdT) by flow cytometry in leukemic disorders. J Histochem Cytochem 1989;37:509–513.

35 Edelman J, Meyerson HJ: Diminished CD3 expression is useful for detecting and enumerating Sezary cells. Am J Clin Pathol 2000;114:467–477.

36 Jamal S, et al: Immunophenotypic analysis of peripheral T-cell neoplasms. A multiparameter flow cytometric approach. Am J Clin Pathol 2001;116:512–526.

37 Lee PS, CN Lin, SS Chuang: Immunophenotyping of angioimmunoblastic T-cell lymphomas by multiparameter flow cytometry. Pathol Res Pract 2003;199:539–545.

38 Dahmoush L, et al: Adult T-cell leukemia/lymphoma: a cytopathologic, immunocytochemical, and flow cytometric study. Cancer 2002;96:110–116.

39 Yokose N, et al: CD20-positive T cell leukemia/lymphoma: case report and review of the literature. Ann Hematol 2001;80:372–375.

40 Jones D, et al: Absence of CD26 expression is a useful marker for diagnosis of T-cell lymphoma in peripheral blood. Am J Clin Pathol 2001;115:885–892.

Flow Cytometry in Fine-Needle Aspiration
Diagnosis of Lymphomas

Chapter 4

B Cell Neoplasms

WHO Histological Classification of B Cell Neoplasms

Mature B Cell Neoplasms
* Chronic lymphocytic leukemia/small lymphocytic lymphoma
* B cell prolymphocytic leukemia
* Lymphoplasmacytic lymphoma
* Splenic marginal zone lymphoma
* Hairy cell leukemia
* Plasma cell myeloma
  Monoclonal gammopathy of undetermined significance
* Solitary plasmacytoma of bone
* Extraosseous plasmacytoma
  Primary amyloidosis
  Heavy chain diseases
* Extranodal marginal zone B cell lymphoma of mucosa-associated lymphoid tissue (MALT lymphoma)
* Nodal marginal zone B cell lymphoma
* Follicular lymphoma
* Mantle cell lymphoma
* Diffuse large B cell lymphoma
* Mediastinal (thymic) large B cell lymphoma
  Intravascular large B cell lymphoma
  Primary effusion lymphoma (see chap. 9 'Extranodal lymphomas')
* Burkitt lymphoma[1]/leukemia[2]
* Lymphomatoid granulomatosis

Precursor B Cell Neoplasm
* Precursor B lymphoblastic leukemia[1]/lymphoma[2]
(* Indicates subtypes described)

Small Lymphocytic Lymphoma/Chronic Lymphocytic Leukemia

Clinical Features
Mostly middle aged to elderly patients. The patients may be asymptomatic but anemia, spleno-hepatomegaly and nodal enlargement are frequently observed. Bone marrow involvement is found in a majority of cases with chronic lymphocytic leukemia (CLL) but not seen in the early phase of small lymphocytic lymphoma (SLL). Rare CLL patients have only nodal involvement at diagnosis.

The clinical course is indolent and the median survival is 7 years. Transformation to high-grade B cell lymphoma (Richters lymphoma) is relatively rare. Approximately 7% of non-Hodgkin lymphomas (NHL) are of the SLL/CLL type [1].

Cytology (fig. 4.1a, b)
The smears are dominated by small lymphocytes (6–12 μm) with round nuclei which have clumped chromatin (cellules grumelées). The cytoplasm is sparse except in the plasmocytoid variant. In most cases, larger cells such as prolymphocytes with a large pale cytoplasm and para-immunoblasts which are of intermediate size with a grey-blue cytoplasm and a large nucleus can be found [2–6]. Incipient transformation is indicated by an increased number of immature cells.

Differential diagnoses: Indolent lymphadenitis, lympho-plasmocytoid lymphoma, CLL of T cell type, follicular lymphoma (low grade), mantle cell lymphoma.

Immunocytochemistry (fig 4.1c, d): The cells are CD19, CD20, CD79a, CD5, CD23 positive. Surface Ig expression is usually weak. A low (<10%) MIB-1 positivity is typical (table 4.1). Higher MIB-1 values indicate an aggressive variant.

Genetics: Trisomy 12, (20%), deletion 13 q (50%), deletion 11 q (20%) (table 4.1).

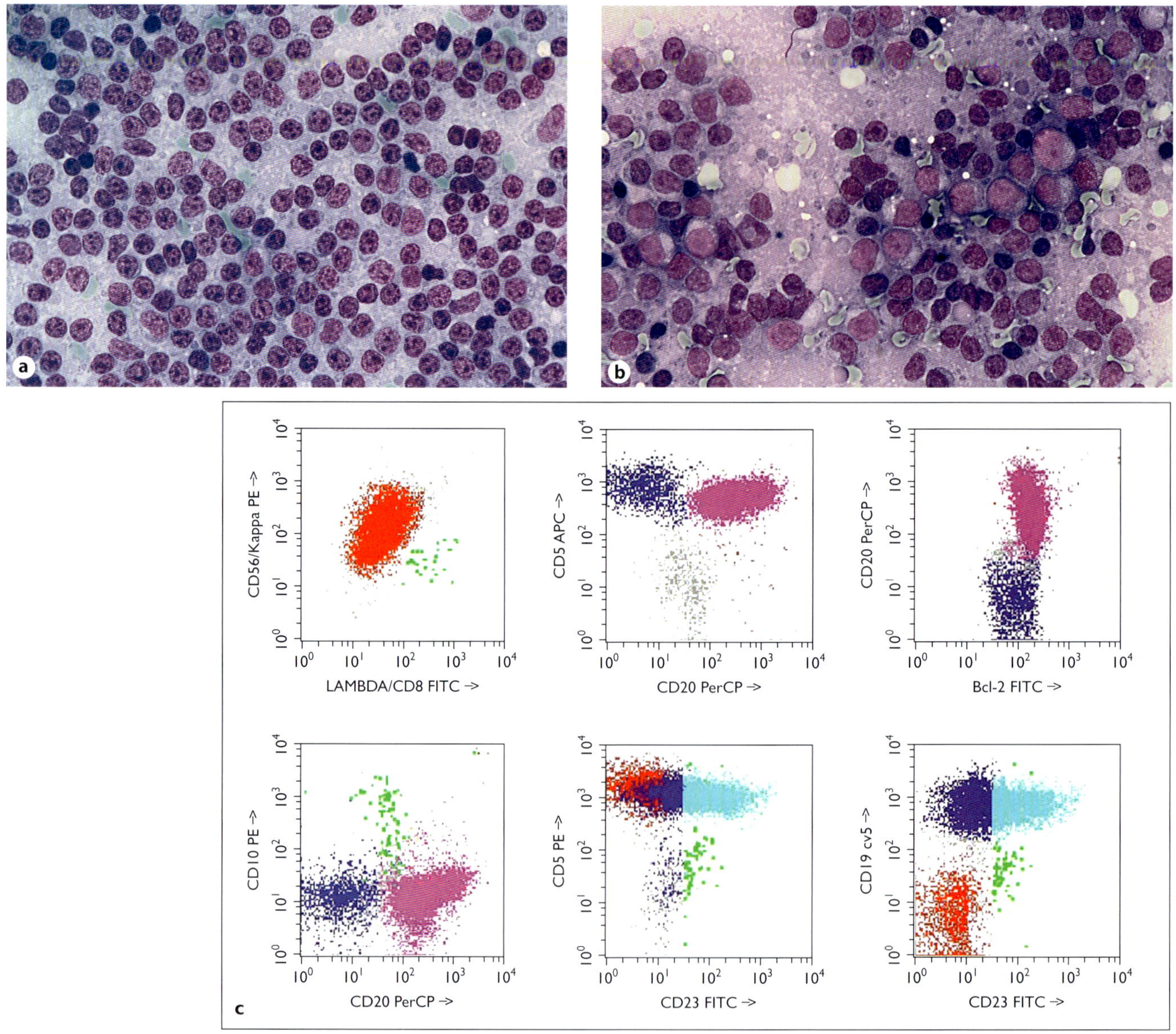

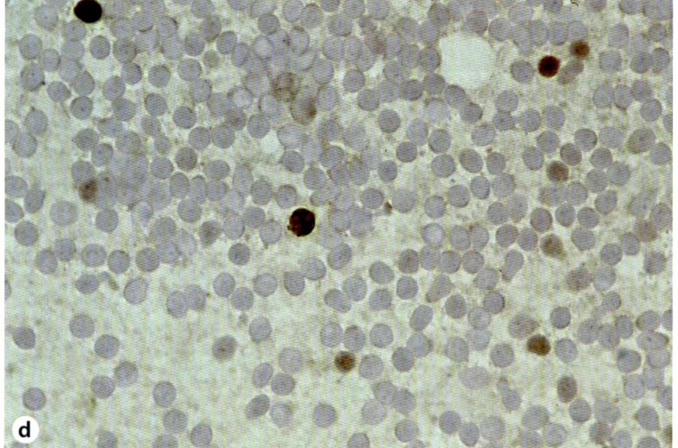

Fig. 4.1. a SLL/ CLL. The aspiration smear is dominated by small lymphocytes. MGG, high-power view. **b** Incipient transformation is shown by an increased number of immature cells. MGG, high-power view. **c** Flow cytometry immunophenotyping of fine needle aspirate from a lymph node with lymphocytic lymphoma of B-CLL type. Four-color flow cytometry was used (for details, see chap. 3). Upper left plot shows a dominance of kappa+ cells within the B cell population (side scatter = gating on CD19: red dots = kappa+ cells; green dots = lambda+ cells). Upper middle plot shows that most CD20+ B cells were positive for CD5 (violet dots). Upper right plot shows that CD20/CD5+ B cells (violet dots) had higher expression of Bcl-2 than CD5+CD20– T cells (blue dots). Lower left plot shows that CD20+ B-cells were negative for CD10 (violet dots), that was positive in a few granulocytes (green dots). Lower middle and right plot illustrate that CD5+ B cells were also partly positive for CD23 (cyan dots). **d** Small lymphocytic lymphoma/chronic lymphocytic leukemia. Few proliferating cells as shown by MIB-1 staining of nuclei. Same case as **a**. Immuno-peroxidase, high-power view.

Table 4.1. Immunologic and genetic characteristics of small-intermediate cell CD20+ B cell lymphomas

Subtype	Immunology	MIB %	Genetics
Small cell lymphocytic	CD5, CD23	<10	trisomy 12
Lymphoplasmacytic	CD43 (+/−)	<5	t(9:14) 50%
Hairy cell leukaemia	CD11c, CD25	<5	−
Marginal zone	CD23 (+/−)	5–30	trisomy 3, t(11; 18)
Follicular	CD10, CD23 (+/−)	5–70	t(14;18)
Mantle cell	CD5, CD43, cyclin D	10–50	t(11;14)

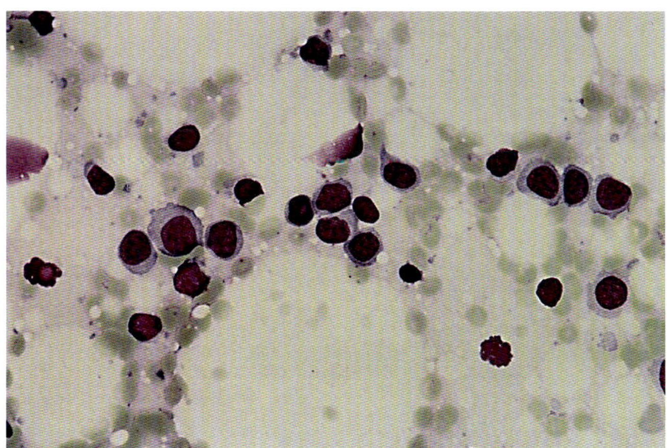

Fig. 4.2. B cell prolymphocytic leukemia. Lymph node aspirate shows medium-sized cells with distinct cytoplasm and poorly defined nucleoli mixed with some mature lymphocytes.

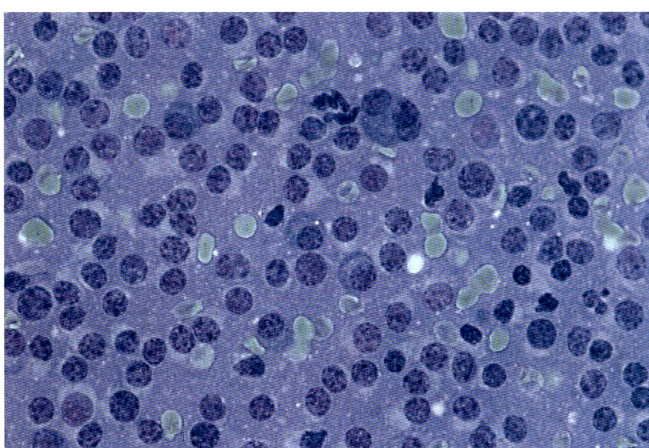

Fig. 4.3. Lymphoplasmacytic lymphoma. Smear from aspirate shows lymphocytes, plasmacytoid cells with eccentric nuclei and some plasma cells. MGG, high-power view.

B Cell Prolymphocytic Leukemia

Clinical Features

This is a distinctly rare disease which is seen in elderly patients. The bone marrow and spleen are involved but lymph nodes may also be affected. All patients have a marked lymphocytosis. Response to chemotherapy is poor and survival is short [7].

Cytology (fig. 4.2)

The tumor cell is medium sized and has a moderate amount of weakly grey-blue cytoplasm. The nucleus is round and often has a large nucleolus.

Differential diagnoses: Mantle cell lymphoma, splenic marginal zone lymphoma and CLL.

Immunocytochemistry: The cells express CD20 and CD79a. CD5 may be present but CD23 is always absent.

Genetics: No constant cytogenetic changes have been reported but p53 abnormalities are seen in over 50% of the cases [8].

Lymphoplasmacytic Lymphoma

Clinical Features

Most patients are aged over 60 years and may present with a variety of symptoms ranging from lymphadenopathy and splenomegaly to autoimmune phenomena, coagulopathy or neuropathy. Bone marrow involvement is common. Monoclonal IgM serum paraprotein is usually present. An indolent course is common and the median 5-year survival is around 50%. Transformation to high-grade neoplasms is rare.

This lymphoma is relatively rare and accounts for 1.5% of NHL [1].

Cytology (fig. 4.3)

The smears typically show small lymphocytes and plasmacytoid cells, which have basophilic cytoplasm and eccentric nuclei. Plasma cells are usually found but if they dominate the smears a diagnosis of plasmacytoma is favored. Immunoblasts are found in low numbers [2–6].

Differential diagnoses: CLL, reactive lymphadenitis.

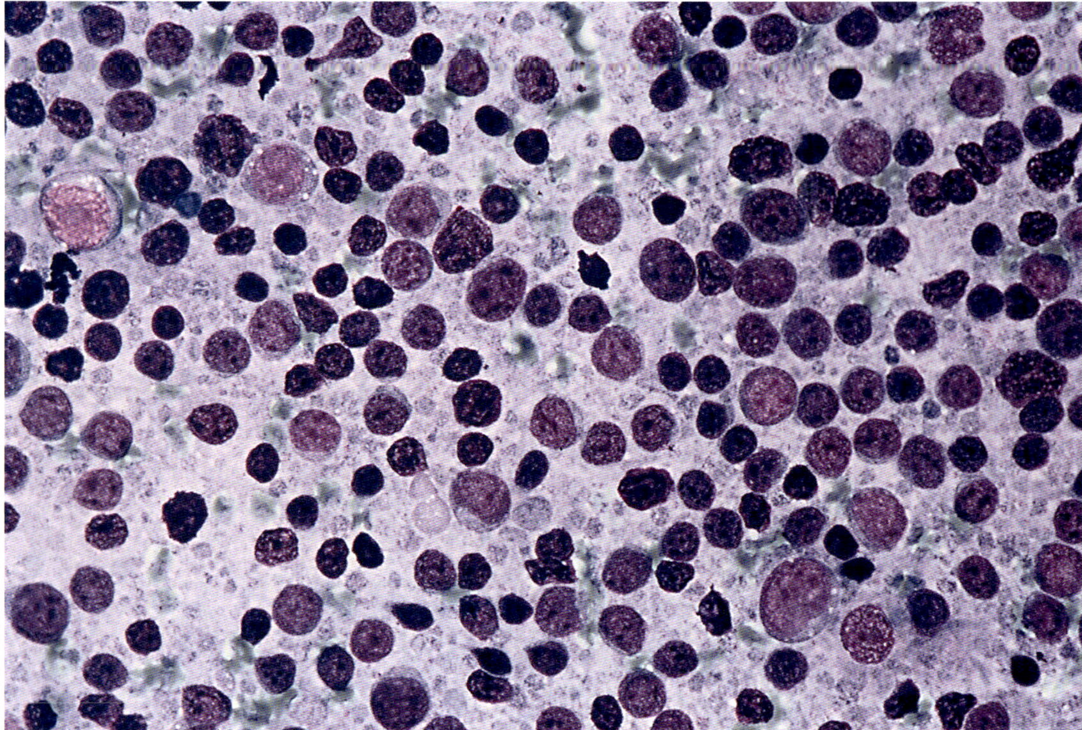

Fig. 4.4. Splenic marginal zone lymphoma. FNA aspirate of the spleen with mixed cell population: small lympho-cytes, medium-sized cells with sparse cytoplasm and few large blasts are found. MGG, high-power view.

Immunocytochemistry: The tumor cells are CD19, CD20, CD38; CD79a positive. CD43 shows variable positivity. CD5 is not expressed. Surface and cytoplasmic Ig staining are positive. The rate of proliferation is often low (<5%) as measured by MIB-1 staining (table 4.1).

Genetics: t (9;14) is seen in 50% of the cases (table 4.1).

Splenic Marginal Zone Lymphoma

Clinical Features
This rare lymphoma affects patients who are middle aged to elderly. Splenomegaly is often the presenting symptom. The bone marrow and liver may be involved but peripheral lymph nodes are often unaffected. This lymphoma often runs an indolent course with a mean survival of around 9 years. The response to chemotherapy is usually poor but splenectomy may result in prolonged survival [9–11].

Cytology (fig. 4.4)
The smears from aspirates of the spleen are dominated by two cell types. One is a small lymphocyte with a round nucleus, dense chromatin and a sparse cytoplasm. The other is a medium-sized cell with a dispersed chromatin and abundant

pale grey-blue cytoplasm. In addition, histiocytes, plasma cells and some larger blastic cells are often present [12].

Differential diagnoses: B-CLL/SLL, mantle cell lymphoma, hairy cell leukemia, and lymphoplasmacytic lymphoma.

Immunocytochemistry: The cells are CD20 and CD79a positive but lack expression of CD5, CD10, CD23, CD43 and CD103. The rate of cell of proliferation is low [9].

Genetics: Allelic loss of chromosome 7q21–32 has been reported in some cases.

Hairy Cell Leukemia

Clinical Features
The patients are middle aged and there is a strong pre-dominance of men. Splenomegaly and opportunistic infec-tions are common symptoms but lymphadenopathy and skin infiltrates can also occur [13]. Long-term remissions are fre-quent after treatment with purine nucleoside analogues.

Cytology (fig. 4.5a)
Smears from lymph nodes or other infiltrates show small- to medium-sized cells with round to oval or bean-shaped nuclei. The cytoplasm is abundant and pale blue. Cytoplasmic

B Cell Neoplasms

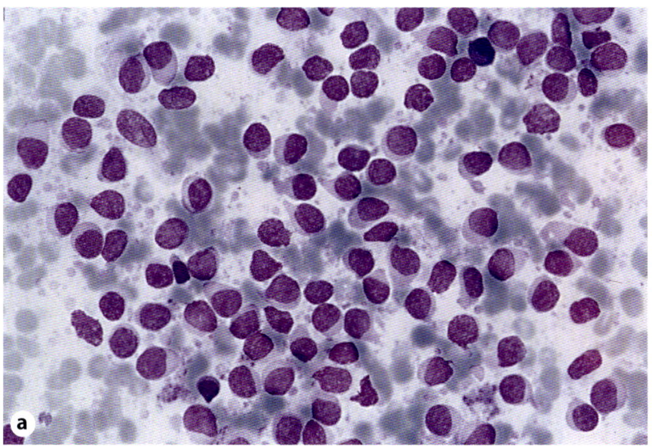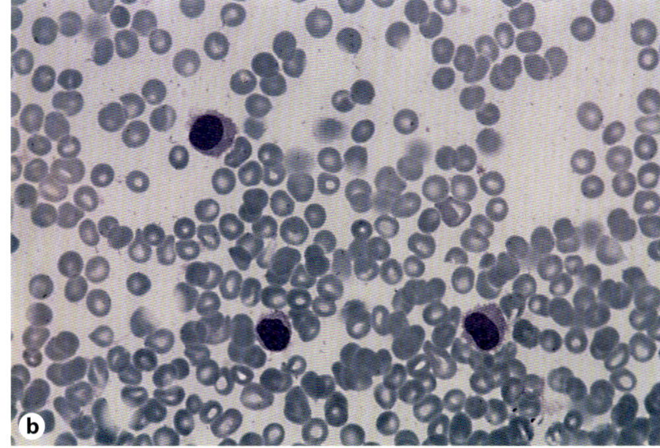

Fig. 4.5. a Hairy cell leukemia. FNA from spleen with monotonous small- to medium-sized cells with eccentric round or oval nuclei and pale blue cytoplasm. **b** Hairy cell leukemia. Peripheral blood smear shows three leukemic cells with typical 'hairy' cytoplasmic projections.

projections typically seen in blood smears (fig. 4.5b) are seldom seen in FNA smears. A conclusive cytologic diagnosis should not be based only on FNA smears from lesions but should be supported by bone marrow findings [14, 15].

Differential diagnosis: CLL, splenic marginal zone lymphoma, lymphoplasmocytic lymphoma, mantle cell lymphoma.

Immunocytochemistry: In addition to C19, CD20 and CD79a, the cells are positive for CD11c, CD25 and CD103. The rate of proliferation is low (table 4.1).

Genetics: No specific abnormality has been described.

Plasma Cell Neoplasms

(1) Myeloma

Clinical Features

Most patients are elderly. The bone marrow is always involved with varying degrees of osteolytic changes. However, extramedullary tumors also occur.

Hypercalcemia, anemia and infections are common symptoms. A M-component can be detected in the serum and urine. The prognosis is usually poor and few patients survive 5 years in spite of intensive therapy. There are, however, indolent variants which can be left untreated for long periods of time [16].

Cytology (fig. 4.6a)

The smears are dominated by plasma cells of varying size. The eccentric nuclei are monomorphic with typically condensed chromatin. Cells with double or multiple nuclei are common. The cytoplasm is typically abundant, grey-blue with a perinuclear lighter-stained area and may contain condensed Ig giving rise to single (Russell bodies) or multiple inclusions

(Mott cells) [2–6, 17]. Some myelomas are immature and the dominating cells are plasmablasts or immunoblast-like cells (fig. 4.6b). Immature blastic and anaplastic variants are uncommon and can be difficult to diagnose using cytomorphology alone (fig. 4.6e, f).

Immunocytochemistry (fig. 4.6c, d): The myeloma/plasmacytoma cells show light chain restriction and express CD38, CD79a and CD138. The pan B antigens CD19 and CD20 are not expressed. The rate of cell proliferation varies between 5–80%.

Genetics: Chromosomal gains and losses are described for a number of chromosomes.

(2) Plasmacytoma (Osseous/Extraosseous)

Clinical Features

The patients are middle aged or elderly. The dominating symptoms are bone pain or fracture for the osseous variant which most often affects vertebrate, ribs and skull. The extraosseous tumors present as localized masses with symptoms related to the site of involvement. A majority of these tumors occur in the nasopharyngeal tract or sinuses. However, lymph node, skin, breast and thyroid may be the primary sites.

These tumors respond well to radiation therapy and the cure rate varies between 40 and 75% for the osseous and extraosseous variants, respectively. In some patients, there is a progression to multiple myeloma [16].

Cytology

The tumor cells are similar to those of myeloma.

Immunocytochemistry: The phenotype expression is similar to that of myeloma.

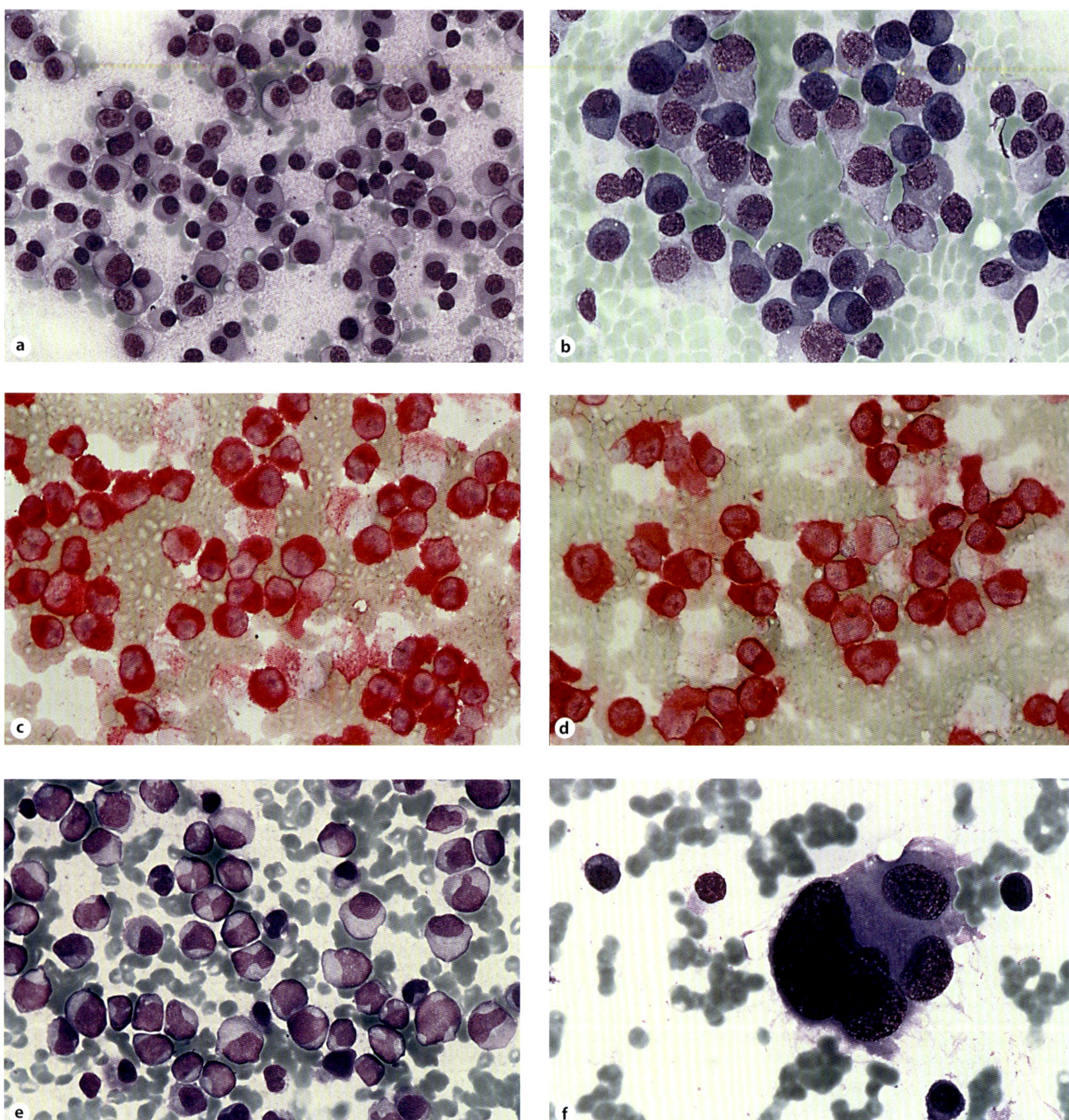

Fig. 4.6. a Myeloma. Smear from aspirate dominated by mature plasma cells of varying size with excentric round nuclei and abundant grey cytoplasm. Few binucleated cells are present. MGG, high-power view. **b** Myeloma. Smear from aspirate with mature plasma cells and large immature plasma cells with round eccentric nuclei with a distinct nucleoli and elongated basophilic cytoplasm. **c** Myeloma. Same case as in **b**, stained positively for kappa light chain showing a monoclonal cell population. Alkaline phosphatase, high-power view. **d** Myeloma. Same case as in **b**, showing positivity of tumor cells for CD138. alkaline phosphatase, high-power view. **e** Anaplastic myeloma. Aspiration smear from blastic variant of myeloma with large pleomorphic cells with irregular nuclei and few plasma cells. MGG, high-power view. **f** Anaplastic myeloma. A bizarre multinucleated cell and few plasma cells. MGG, high-power view.

B Cell Neoplasms

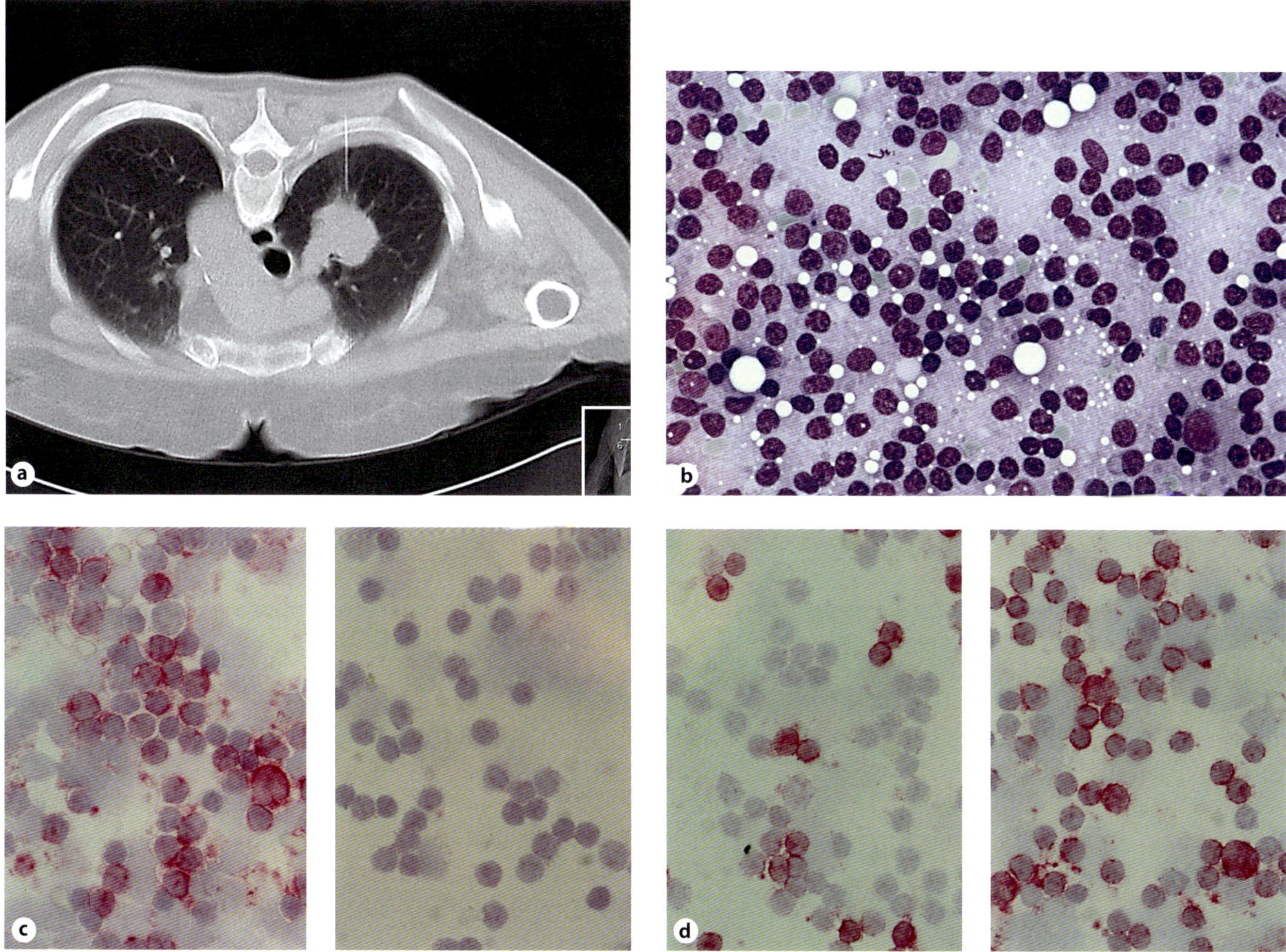

Fig. 4.7. a MALT lymphoma. CT guided FNA of MALT lymphoma in the lung. Courtesy of Dr. Veli Söderlund, Clinical Radiology, Karolinska University Hospital. b. Marginal zone lymphoma. FNA smear shows monomorphic small to medium sized tumor cells. MGG, high-power view. c Immunocytochemistry performed on cytospin preparation from the same case as in b showing kappa+ monoclonal cells (left) and lambda− cells (right). Alkaline phosphatase, high-power view. d Immunostaining with CD3 (left) and IgM expression of tumor cells (right) from the same case as in b.

Marginal Zone Lymphoma/Extranodal (MALT) and Nodal

Clinical Features (fig. 4.7a)

The patients are usually middle aged to elderly. The extranodal (MALT) subtype involves glandular epithelium of various organs. The gastrointestinal tract accounts for 50% of the cases with the stomach being the most frequent site. Other common sites are salivary glands, lung, orbital adnexae, skin, breast and thyroid. Multifocal disease is relatively common. The symptoms range from a palpable mass to functional impairment. Spread to the bone marrow is seen in 1/5 of cases.

There is a rare nodal variant of MALT lymphoma with no extranodal or splenic manifestations.

The clinical course is typically indolent and often preceded by autoimmune disorders or even infections. Local treatment often suffices. Transformation to diffuse large B cell lymphoma can occur [18, 19].

The MALT lymphomas represent approximately 8% of NHL.

Cytology (fig. 4.7b)

The dominating lymphoma cell is small to medium sized with an irregular nucleus (centrocyte-like) and a small nucleolus. The chromatin is coarse and in some cases the pale relatively abundant cytoplasm imparts a monocytoid appearance. A plasmacytic differentiation may also be seen. Monocytes and tingible body macrophages are identified in a majority of cases. Centroblasts, immunoblasts and plasma cells are often present in low numbers [3, 20–22].

Differential diagnoses: Reactive lymphadenitis, follicular lymphoma, mantle cell lymphoma.

Immunocytochemistry (fig. 4.7c, d): The tumor cells are CD20, CD79a, CD21 and CD35 positive. CD43 is variable. Ig expression is seen in all cases. The cells typically lack CD5, CD10 and CD23 (table 4.11). The rate of cell proliferation is highly variable.

Genetics: Trisomy 3 (60%) or t(11;18) (25–50%) (table 4.1).

Follicular Lymphomas

Clinical Features

This lymphoma typically affects middle-aged patients. Widespread lymphadenopathy, both peripheral and central, is the most common symptom but fatigue may dominate. The lymph nodes are involved from the beginning but spread to bone marrow and spleen is common. In advanced stages, involvement of extranodal tissue such as skin and soft tissue is frequently seen.

The clinical course is variable depending on stage and grade but cure is rare. Transformation to high-grade lymphoma is seen in 1/3 of the cases which then have a poor prognosis.

In western countries, follicular lymphomas represent approximately 1/3 of all NHL [1].

Cytology (fig. 4.8)

These tumors show at least two types of neoplastic lymphocytes, the centrocyte and the centroblast (fig. 4.8a). In addition, there is often an admixture of small reactive lymphocytes of T phenotype. Histiocytes of epitheloid type may be numerous in some cases.

The centrocytes vary in size between different tumors but the individual cell has a rounded nucleus with a narrow rim of pale blue cytoplasm (MGG). The nucleus is characteristically cleaved, sometimes to the extent that it looks bi-lobed. Nucleoli are rarely seen.

The second tumor cell, the centroblast, is medium sized to large and has a round nucleus with a reticular chromatin pattern. One to several usually small nucleoli can be observed and they are often located at the nuclear membrane (fig. 4.8b). The cytoplasm is moderately abundant, stains blue and frequently has vacuoles [2–6, 23, 24]. A special variant of this lymphoma is the signet-ring cell variant (fig. 4.8c). The proportion of centroblasts varies among cases and there seems to be a correlation between increasing number of centroblasts and poor clinical outcome. A 3-grading system has been recommended for histopathology based on high-power microscopic field counting of the number of centroblasts in ten neoplastic follicles (fig. 4.8d, e). Thus, grades 1, 2 and 3 cases have 0–5, 6–15 and >15 centroblasts per high-power field, respectively [6]. A similar grading can be done on smears calculating the percentage of centroblasts [24].

However, we have found that analysis of the fraction of proliferating centrocytes and centroblasts is more reproducible. In our series, this figure varies between 5 and 70% (table 4.1). Based on this, we suggest that grades 1, 2 and 3 correspond to a proliferation fraction of <15, 15–30 and >30%, respectively (fig. 4.8f).

Differential diagnoses: Reactive lymphadenitis, mantle cell lymphoma, diffuse large B-cell lymphoma.

Immunocytochemistry (fig 4.8g): The tumor cells are monoclonal and CD19, CD20, CD79a and CD10 positive. bcl-2 is expressed in most cases. CD5 and CD43 are not expressed. The proliferating fraction varies between 5 and 70% (table 4.1).

Genetics (fig 4.8h): t (14;18) is observed in up to 95% of the cases (table 4.1).

Mantle Cell Lymphoma

Clinical Features

The patients are most often elderly. Lymphadenopathy, splenohepatomegaly, lymphocytosis, anemia and fatigue are the most common symptoms. In addition to lymph nodes, spleen, liver and bone marrow, the gastrointestinal tract is commonly involved.

The median survival is less than 5 years and cure is rarely observed. Transformation to a blastoid lymphoma seems to be relatively frequent.

Mantle cell lymphomas comprise approximately 7% of NHL [1].

Cytology (fig. 4.9a)

The smears are dominated by small-medium sized tumor cells which resemble centrocytes with a sparse weakly basophilic cytoplasm. The nucleus has an irregular contour with dispersed chromatin and discrete nucleoli. Epitheloid histiocytes and plasma cells are frequently seen [3–6, 24, 26–28].

The blastic variant has intermediate- to large-sized cells with round nuclei, dispersed chromatin, and mitoses are easily seen (fig. 4.9b) [29].

Differential diagnoses: Follicular lymphoma, marginal cell lymphoma, large B cell lymphoma.

Immunocytochemistry (fig. 4.9c): The cells are monoclonal and CD5, CD19, CD20, CD43 positive. All cases express bcl-2 and cyclin D1 (fig. 4.9d). CD10 and CD23 are

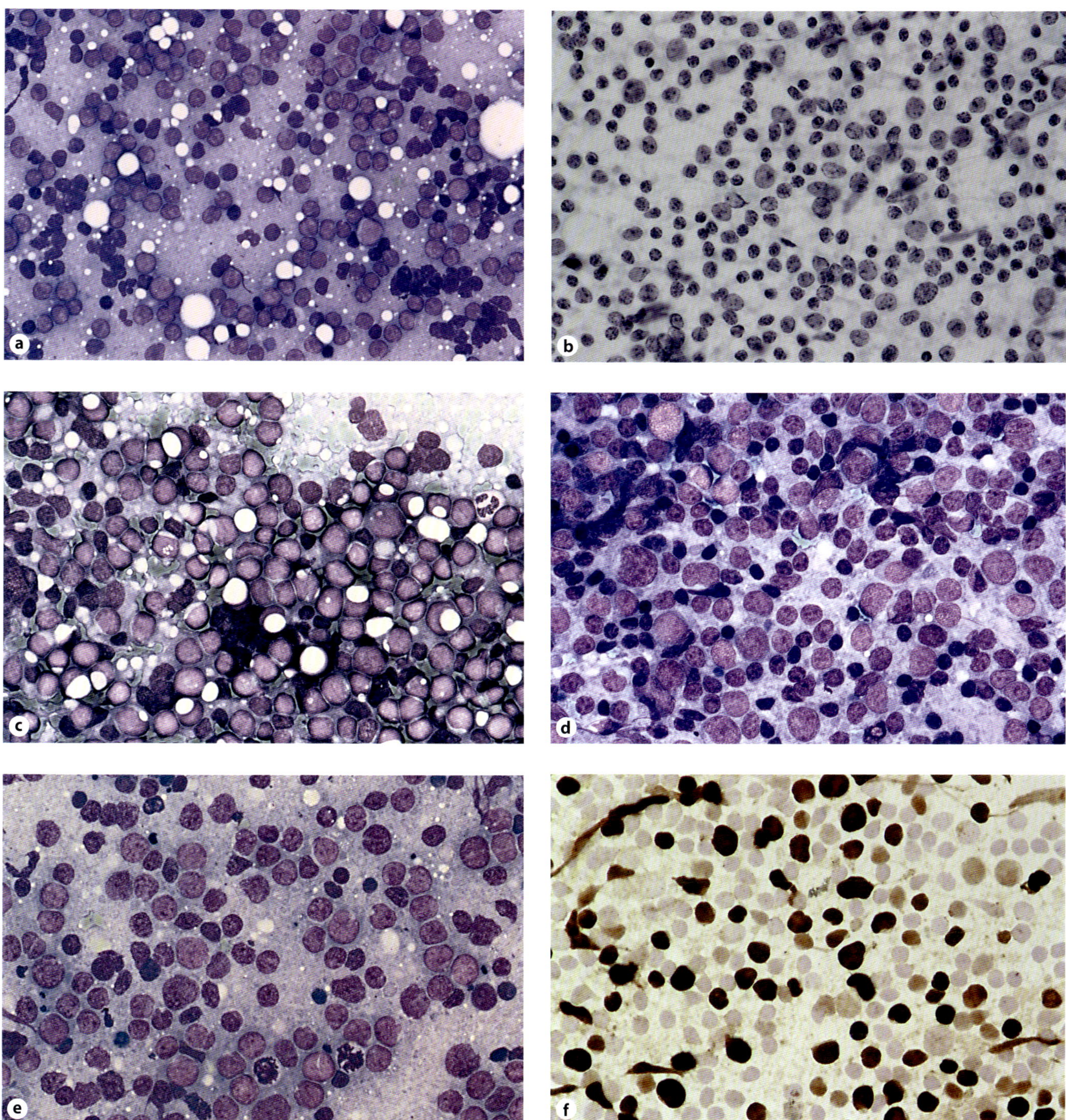

Fig. 4.8. a Follicular lymphoma grade 1. FNA smear shows mixture of small, medium and large-sized lymphoid cells. The dominating small- to medium-sized cells have irregular nuclei and sparse cytoplasm. MGG, high-power view. **b** Follicular lymphoma grade 1. Mixed cell population with dominance of small- to medium-sized cells. Papanicolaou, high-power view. **c** Follicular lymphoma grade 1. Large cytoplasmic vacuoles in some of the cells results in a signet-ring variant. MGG, high-power view. **d** Follicular lymphoma grade 2. FNA smear showing higher proportion of centroblasts as compared to grade 1. MGG, high-power view. **e** Follicular lymphoma grade 3. FNA smear presenting predominance of immature blasts with round nuclei. MGG, high-power view. **f** Follicular lymphoma grade 2. Proliferating cells showed by brown nuclei in approximately 30% of cells with MIB-1 staining. Immunoperoxidase, high-power view.

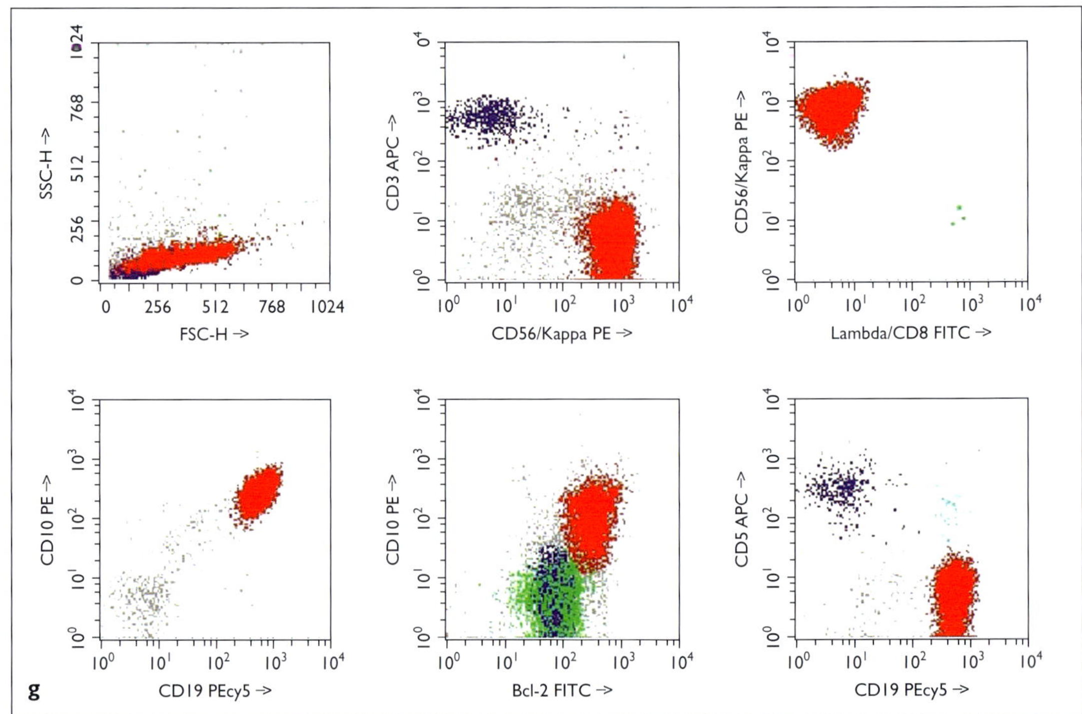

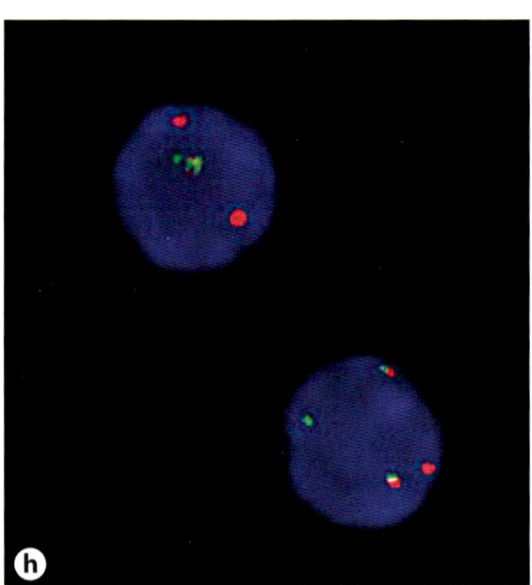

Fig. 4.8. g Flow cytometry immunophenotyping of fine-needle aspirate from a lymph node with follicular lymphoma. Four-color flow cytometry was used. Upper left plot shows forward scatter/side scatter image of the sample with kappa+ B cells (red dots) being larger in size than CD3+ T lymphocytes (blue dots). Upper middle plot shows that kappa+ B cells (red dots) are much more numerous than CD3+ T cells (blue dots). Upper right plot shows a dominance of kappa+ within the B cell population (side scatter = gating on CD19–; red dots = kappa+ cells; green dots = lambda+ cells). Lower left plot shows that most B cells were positive for CD10 (red dots). Lower middle plot illustrates that CD10+ B cells had high expression of Bcl-2 (red dots) as compared with CD5+ T cells (green dots) and CD10– B-cells (blue dots). Lower right plot shows that most B cells (red dots) were negative for CD5. CD5 was positive in T cells (blue dots) and a minor population of B cells from mantle zones (cyan dots). **h** Follicular lymphoma. Vysis LSI IGH/BCL2 Dual Color, Dual Fusion Translocation Probe, detecting the translocation t(14;18)(q32;q21). In the normal cell (top) two red (BCL2) and two green (IGH) signals can be seen. In the tumor cell (low) the translocation splits the two genes and creates two red/green fusion signals. Courtesy of Dr. E Blennow, Clinical Genetics, Karolinska University Hospital.

not expressed. The MIB-1 index varies between 10 and 50% (table 4.1). In the blastic variant, it is not uncommon to find over 90% of the cells in proliferation (fig. 4.9e).

Genetics (fig. 4.9f): t (11;14) occurs in almost all cases (table 4.1).

Diffuse Large B Cell Lymphoma

Clinical Features

The median age of patients is in the 7th decade, but young adults and children are occasionally affected. The dominating symptom is that of a rapidly enlarging mass. The lymph nodes are often engaged but extranodal spread (soft tissue, bone, CNS, lung) is not uncommon. In fact, extranodal tumors can be the primary presentation.

This is a highly aggressive group of lymphomas which, however, is potentially curable.

Almost 40% of all NHL are of this subtype [1].

Cytology (fig. 4.10)

This group of tumors has an extremely variable morphologic appearance. One type is composed of monomorphic typical centroblasts with few other cells present (fig. 4.10a).

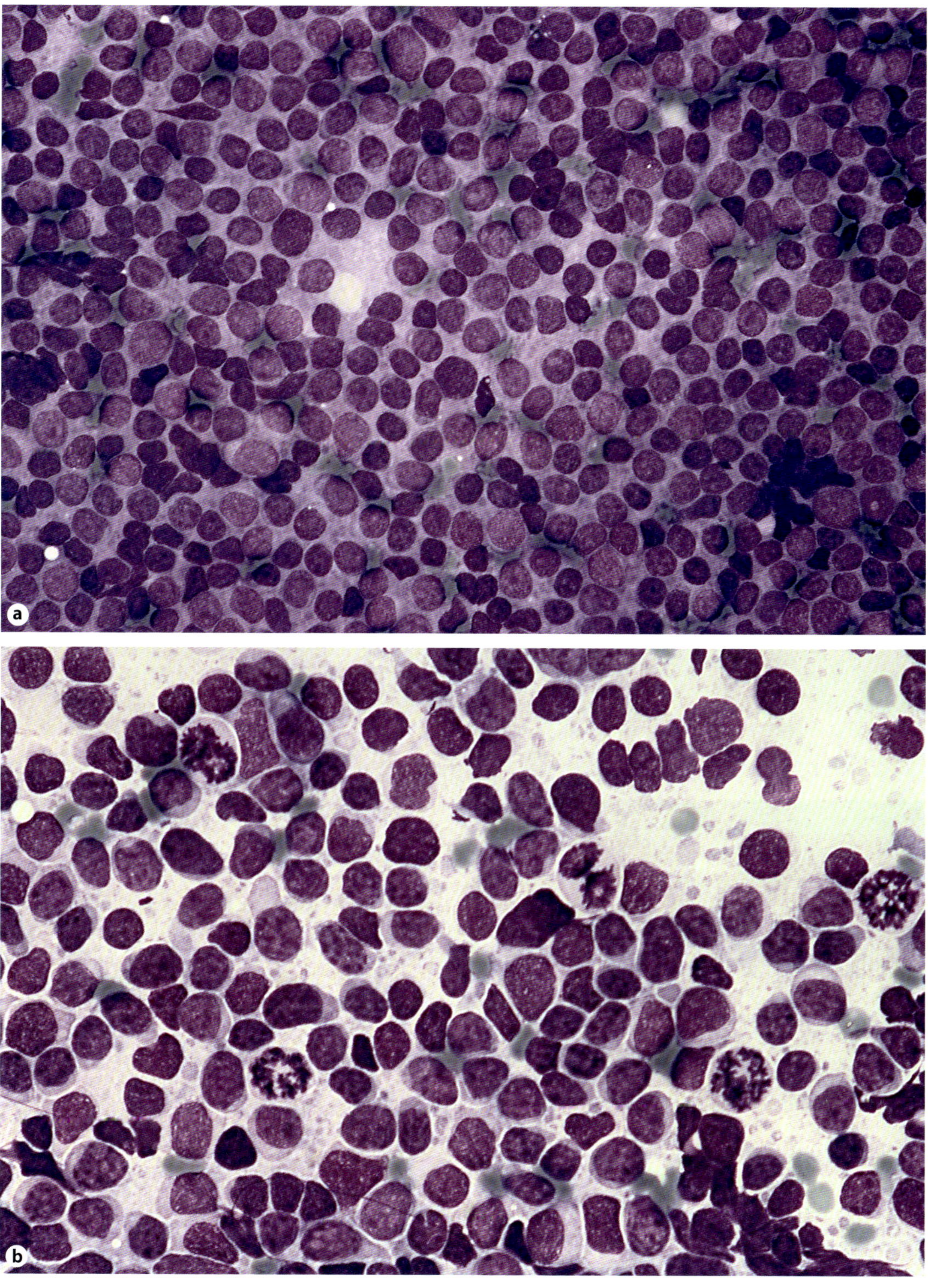

Fig. 4.9. **a** Mantle cell lymphoma. FNA smear showing small-medium sized tumor cells with irregular often cleaved nuclei. MGG, high-power view. **b** Mantle cell lymphoma, blastic variant. The aspirated material shows tumor cells of intermediate to large size. Numerous mitotic figures. MGG, high-power view.

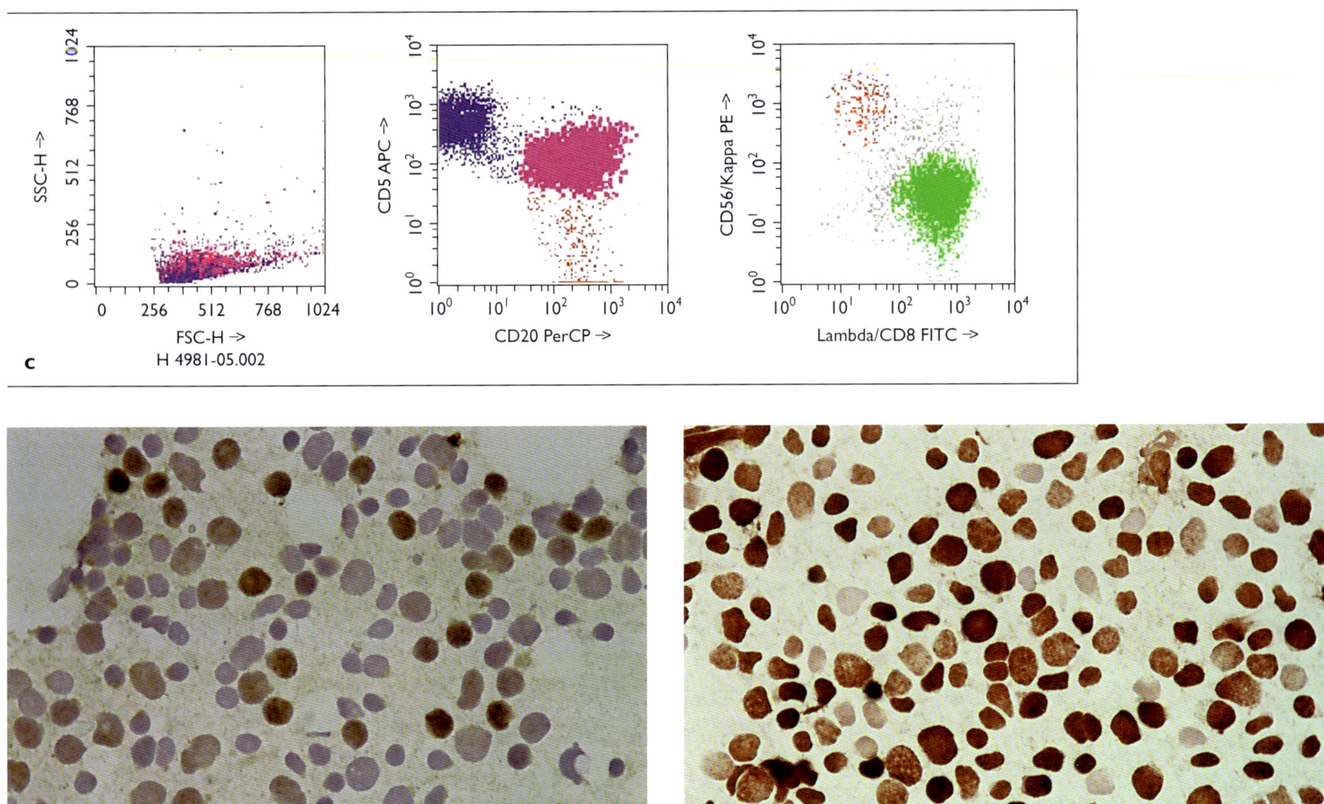

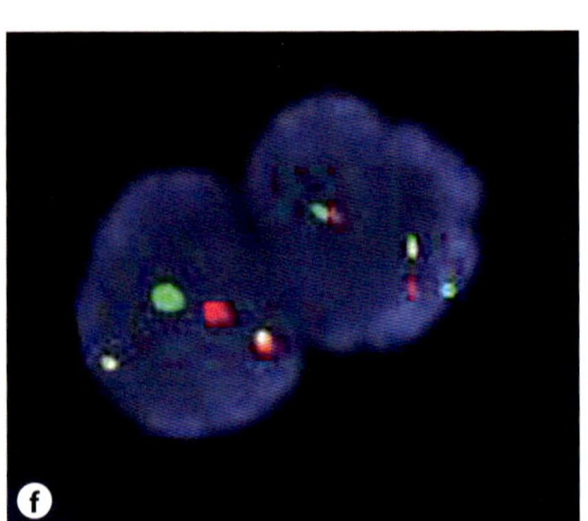

Fig. 4.9. c Mantle cell lymphoma. Flow cytometry immunophenotyping of fine-needle aspirate from a lymph node with mantle cell lymphoma. Four-color flow cytometry was used. Left plot shows forward scatter/side scatter image of the sample with CD5+/CD20+ B cells (violet dots) being larger in size than CD5+/CD20− T lymphocytes (blue dots). Middle plot shows that most B cells were positive for CD5. Right plot shows a dominance of lambda+ cells within the B cell population (side scatter = gating on CD19-; red dots = kappa+ cells; green dots = lambda+ cells). **d** Mantle cell lymphoma. Cyclin D1-positive tumor cells mixed with negative mature lymphocytes. Immunoperoxidase, high-power view. **e**. Mantle cell lymphoma, blastic variant. Immunostaining with MIB-1, shows over 90% positive cells. Immunoperoxidase, high-power view. **f**. Mantle cell lymphoma. Interphase FISH on tumor cells using Vysis LSI IGH/CCNDI Dual Color, Dual Fusion Translocation Probe, detecting the translocation t(11;14)(q13;q32). In a normal cell, two red (CCNDI) and two green (IGH) signals can be seen (not shown). In the two tumor cells, the translocation splits the two genes and creates two red/green fusion signals. Courtesy of Dr. E. Blennow, Clinical Genetics, Karolinska University Hospital.

A second type is composed of centroblasts and a varying number of immunoblasts (fig. 4.10b). True immunoblastic cases are also found but much less frequently. Other types include large cells with cleaved or multilobated nuclei which often have a finely granular chromatin (fig. 4.10c, d). These cells are fragile and often stripped of their cytoplasm in smears. When present it is pale grey-blue and abundant. These variants may be difficult to recognize as of lymphoid origin even in MGG-stained smears (fig. 4.10e). The rare large B cell anaplastic lymphoma is also included in this subgroup. Irrespective of its name this variant seems to have a lesser degree of cellular anaplasia than its counterpart on the T cell side [2–6, 30]. Finally, T cell-rich B cell lymphoma (TCRBCL) has been assigned to this subgroup. Smears from this rare type are dominated (>90%) by small mature reactive T lymphocytes and only few large tumor cells can be found (fig. 4.10f). The tumor cells may mimic Hodgkin's cells but most often look like large centroblasts [31, 32]. Rare

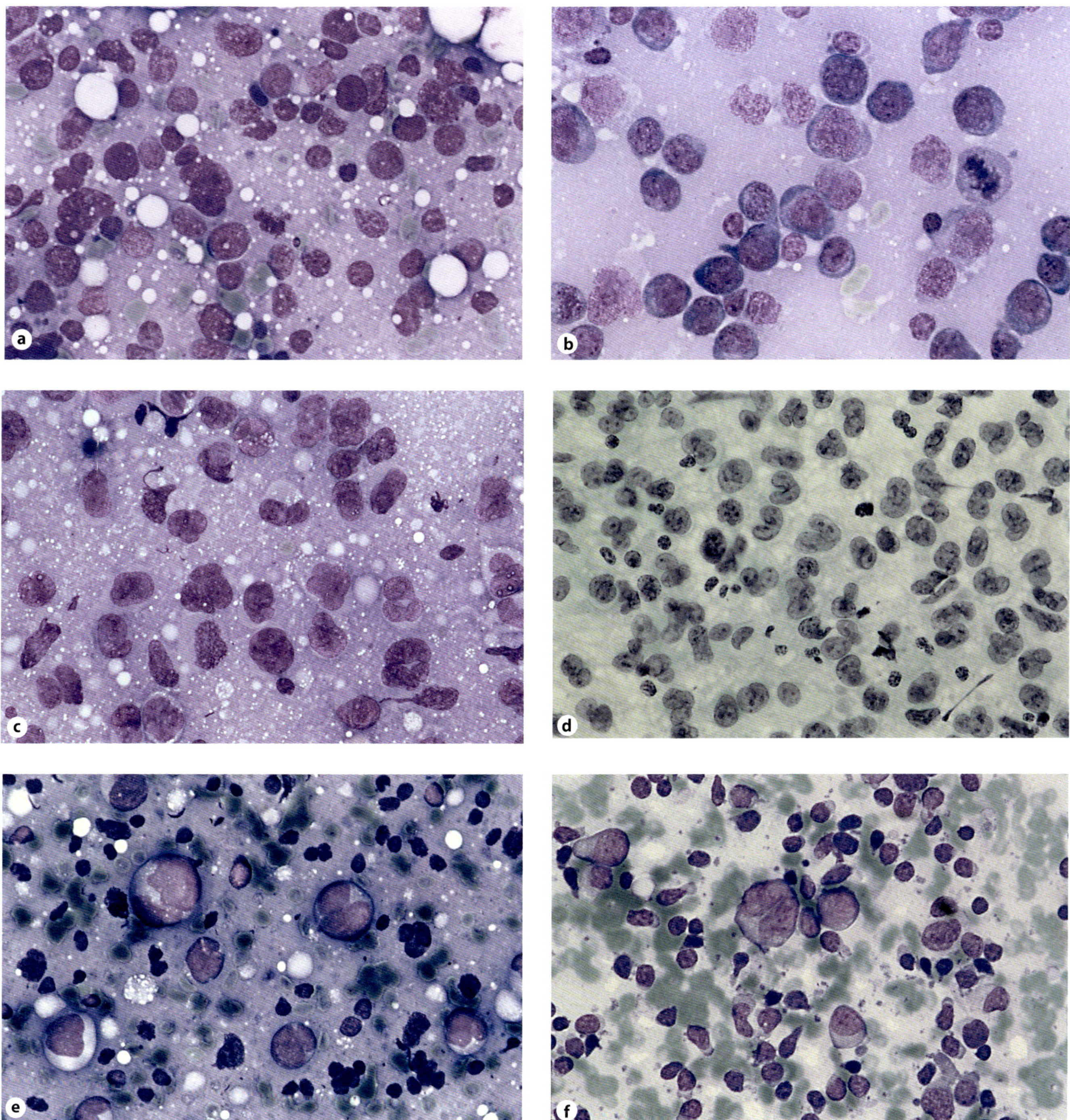

Fig. 4.10. a Diffuse large B cell lymphoma. FNA smear with monomorphic centroblasts. MGG, high-power view. **b** Diffuse large B cell lymphoma. Smear with large immunoblasts of markedly varying sizes, round nuclei with coarse chromatin and distinctly basophilic cytoplasm. MGG, high-power view. **c** Diffuse large B cell lymphoma. Pleomorphic large lymphoma cells some with multilobated nuclei. MGG, high-power view. **d** Diffuse large B cell lymphoma. The extreme pleomorphism of the nuclei is clearly demonstrated in the Papanicoulaou-stained smear. The same case as in figure 6.10c. **e** Diffuse large B cell lymphoma. Poorly differentiated tumor cells with lobated and cleaved nuclei. MGG, high-power view. **f**. T cell-rich B cell lymphoma. The smear is dominated by small mature lymphocytes of T phenotype with few large polymorphic tumor cells. One binucleated cell which mimics a Reed-Sternberg cell. MGG, high-power view.

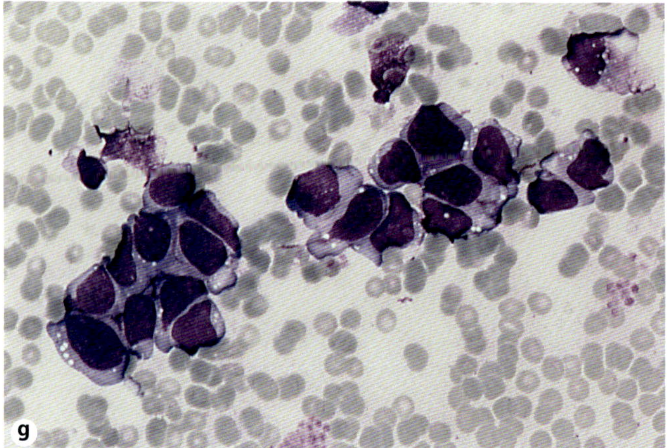

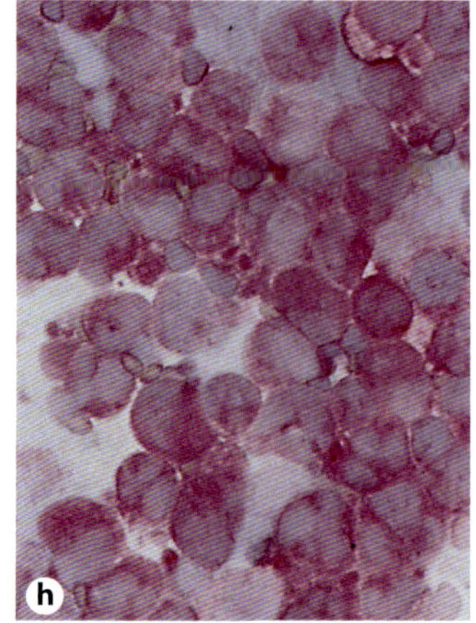

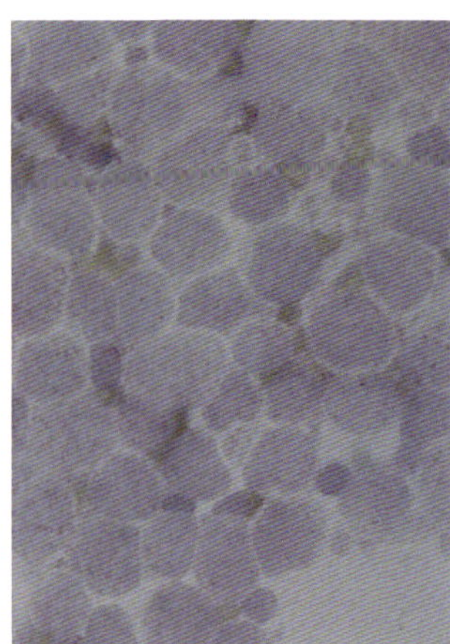

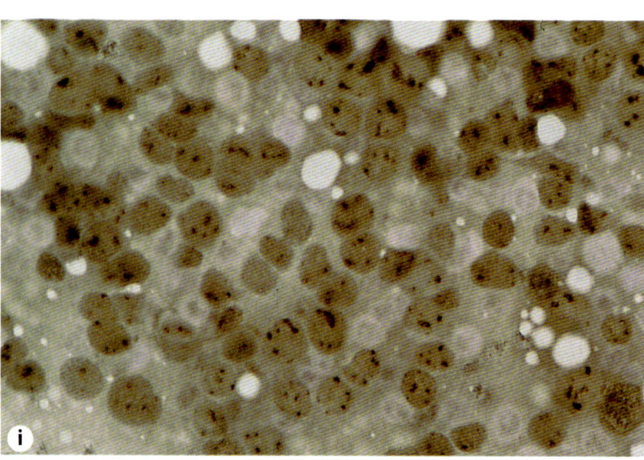

Fig. 4.10. g Diffuse large B cell lymphoma. Immature lymphoma cells with a large vacuolated cytoplasm and cohesive tendency mimicking poorly differentiated cancer. MGG, high-power view. **h** Diffuse large B cell lymphoma. Immunocytochemistry on cytospin preparation from the same aspirate as in **a** showing monoclonal kappa+ (left) and lambda− cells. Alkaline phosphatase, high-power view. **i** Diffuse large B cell lymphoma. High number of MIB-1-positive cells showing distinct nucleoli of centroblasts. Immunoperoxidase, high-power view.

cases of large cell lymphoma may mimic carcinoma (fig. 4.10g).

Differential diagnosis: Extreme reactive follicular hyperplasia, follicular lymphoma (grade 3), blastic variant of mantle cell lymphoma, poorly differentiated carcinomas and seminoma.

Immunocytochemistry (fig. 4.10h): The cells are monoclonal and CD19, CD20 and CD79a positive. Expression of CD10 is seen in the centroblastic variant and CD30 in the large cell anaplastic tumors. Bcl2 and bcl6 are frequently expressed. The rate of proliferation as measured by the MIB-1 index is above 50% (fig. 4.10i).

Genetics: t(14;18) is observed in 1/3 of the cases.

Mediastinal Large B Cell Lymphoma

Clinical Features

The patients are middle aged and there is a female predominance. The symptoms relate to a large mediastinal mass with shortness of breath and venous stasis in patients with localized disease. Mediastinal lymph nodes are involved by definition, but extranodal sites (skin, liver, brain) may also become affected. This is an aggressive lymphoma which may be cured in the early stages. Disseminated disease has a poor prognosis.

Cytology (fig. 4.11)

The smears are dominated by large pleomorphic cells with a pale abundant cytoplasm. Eosinophils are present in small numbers. Fragments of collagen are found as well as small benign lymphocytes. Fibrosis may result in scanty smears [30, 33, 34].

Differential diagnosis: Hodgkin lymphoma, diffuse large B cell lymphoma.

Immunocytochemistry: The tumor cells are monoclonal and CD19, CD20, and often weakly CD30 positive. CD5 and CD10 are not expressed. In addition, the cells are CD45 positive, which distinguishes them from Hodgkin cells. The rate of proliferation is over 50%.

Genetics: So far, no constant aberrations have been described.

B Cell Neoplasms

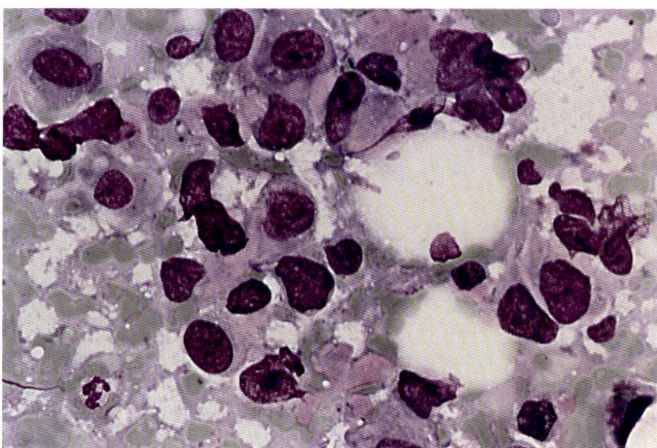

Fig. 4.11. Mediastinal B cell lymphoma. Large pleomorphic cells with pale abundant cytoplasm with small vacuoles and irregular nuclei with coarse chromatin. Small collagen fragments are seen. MGG, high-power view.

Burkitt Lymphoma

Clinical Features

Three clinical variants exist: the endemic (in Africa), the sporadic (found in Europe and USA) and the HIV-associated type. Facial bone involvement, particularly the jaws, is commonly seen in the endemic type. Sporadic cases often present with ileocecal or retroperitoneal masses while the HIV type commonly presents with lymphadenopathy. However, all types have a high risk for CNS, ovary, breast and kidney involvement. Most patients present with large tumors but few present with bone marrow involvement. With intensive chemotherapy cure is expected in a majority of the patients.

Cytology (fig 4.12a)

The smears are dominated by medium-sized tumor cells with many macrophages interspersed. The lymphoblasts have slightly irregular nuclei with coarse chromatin and distinct, small nucleoli. The cytoplasm is typically deeply basophilic and has several small vacuoles. Mitotic figures are numerous. An atypical variant of Burkitt lymphoma exists, which shows greater variation in nuclear size and shape [2–6, 35–39].

Differential diagnosis: Lymphoblastic lymphoma of B or T origin, granulocytic sarcoma.

Immunocytochemistry: The tumor cells are monoclonal and express CD10, CD19 and CD20. They typically lack TdT and BCL2. The proliferation rate is close to 100% as measured by MIB-1 staining (fig. 4.12b).

Genetics: Most cases have a (8;14) translocation (fig. 4.12c) but t(2;8) or t(8;22) can also exist.

Lymphomatoid Granulomatosis

Clinical Features

This is a rare EBV-driven disorder which can occur at any age. Most patients are immunodeficient either because of treatment, HIV infection or genetic predisposition. The lungs are commonly involved but brain, liver and skin are other frequent sites. The lymph nodes are rarely affected. Cough, dyspnea, fever and malaise are common symptoms. The prognosis is variable and related to the numbers of EBV-positive immature B cells with grade 1 showing only occasional transformed B cells and grade 3 dominated by the transformed cells. Spontaneous regression or response to interferon can be seen in cases with grades 1 and 2. Grade 3 lesions require aggressive therapy [40].

Cytology

The tumor cells may mimic immunoblasts but can be pleomorphic or Hodgkin-like or even mimic carcinoma. There is a background of necrosis, mature lymphoid cells, plasma cells and histiocytes [40–42].

Immunocytochemistry: The atypical cells are CD20 and LMP-1 positive. They are variably positive for CD30 and CD79a. Monoclonal light chain expression is rare.

Genetics: PCR can demonstrate clonality of the immunoglobulin genes.

Precursor B Lymphoblastic Leukemia/Lymphoma

Clinical Features

A majority of lymphoma patients are under 18 years of age, while children with leukemia are under 6 years. Patients with lymphoma often show lymph node, skin and bone involvement. The symptoms are palpable masses or bone pain. The leukemic patients present with bone marrow failure in a majority of cases, but bone pain is also common.

With present chemotherapy, the prognosis for B-ALL is relatively good but young patients (<1 year) and cases with t(9;22) or t(4;11) have a worse prognosis. Lymphoma patients respond well to chemotherapy but the long-term prognosis is relatively poor.

Cytology (fig. 4.13a)

The cells are small to medium sized and relatively monomorphus but some variation in size is not uncommon. The nuclei are round and often convoluted. The chromatin is finely granular and small nucleoli are common. The sparse cytoplasm may contain small azurophilic granules. Mitoses are numerous [2–6, 43–46].

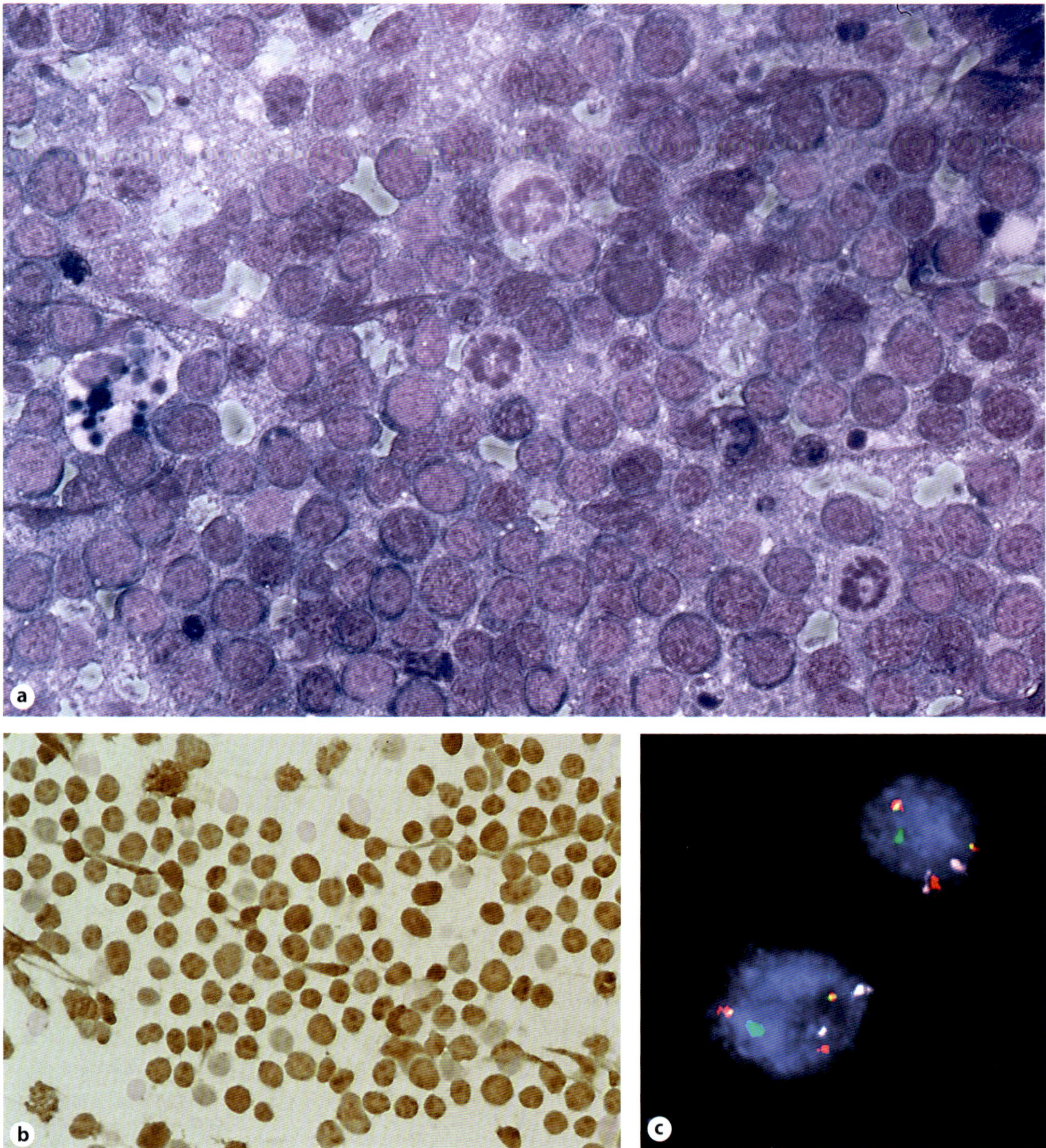

Fig. 4.12. a Burkitt lymphoma. Smear shows dominance of medium sized lymphoblasts with scanty heavily basophilic cytoplasm. Mitotic figures are easily identified. One macrophage with cytoplasmic apoptotic fragments. MGG, high-power view. **b** Burkitt lymphoma. MIB-1-stained smear shows that almost all cells are proliferating. Immunoperoxidase, high-power view. **c** Burkitt lymphoma. Interphase FISH on tumor cells using Vysis LSI IGH/MYC, CEP 8 Tri-color , Dual Color, Dual Fusion Translocation Probe, detecting the translocation t(8;14) (q24;q32). In a normal cell, two red (MYC), two green (IGH) and two purple (centromere 8) signals can be seen (not shown). In the two tumor cells, the translocation splits the two genes and creates two red/green fusion signals. The centromere probe serves as control for possible MYC amplification and loss of der(8). Courtesy of Dr. E. Blennow, Clinical Genetics, Karolinska University Hospital.

B Cell Neoplasms

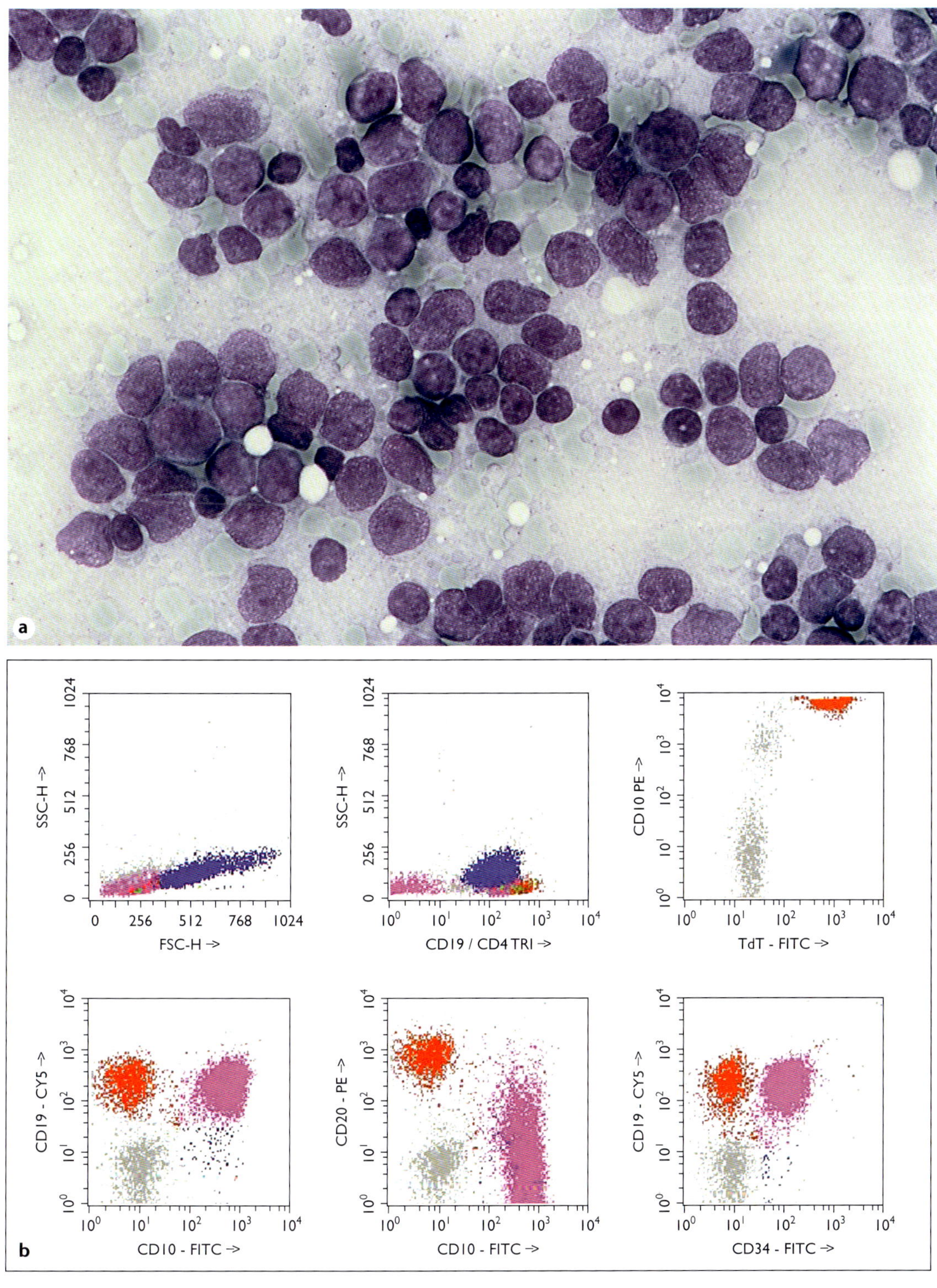

Fig. 4.13. a Precursor B-LB/ALL. Smear with dominance of medium sized immature blasts with irregular nuclei and sparse cytoplasm. MGG,high-power field. **b** B precursor ALL. Flow cytometry immunophenotyping of fine-needle aspirate from a lymph node with a B precursor acute lymphoblastic leukemia. Four-color flow cytometry was used. Screening showed a population of CD19+ cells that had scatter characteristics of blasts (upper left and middle plot, blue dots) and were negative for immunoglobulin light chains (not shown). Additional staining for TdT/CD10/CD19 (right upper plot red dots, left lower plot violet dots) showed overexpression of CD10 together with positivity for Tdt. The cells were negative for CD20 as shown in the lower middle plot (violet dots) and positive for CD34 (right lower plot, violet dots).

Differential diagnosis: Burkitt and Burkitt-like lymphoma, granulocytic sarcoma.

Immunocytochemistry: The lymphoblasts are positive for CD19, CD79a as well as TdT. Most cases express CD10 and CD20 but CD45 may be absent (fig. 4.13b). The MIB-1 index is high (>50%).

Genetics: Several abnormalities have been described in the blasts from ALL as well as LBL. Hypo-, hyper- or pseudodiploid cases as well as those with translocations (9:22), (12:21) or (1:19) seem to be the most frequently described alterations.

References

1 Anon: A clinical evaluation of the International Lymphoma Study Group classification of non-Hodgkin's lymphoma. The non-Hodgkin's Lymphoma Classification Project. Blood 1997;89:3903–3918.

2 Das D: Lymph nodes; in Bibbo M (ed): Comprehensive Cytopathology, ed 2. Philadelphia, Saunders, 1997, pp 703–731.

3 Bizjak-Schwarzbartl M: Color Atlas of Non-Hodgkin's Lymphoma: Fine Needle Aspiration Biopsy. Ljubljana, Institute of Oncology, 1994.

4 Skoog L, Tani E: Lymph nodes; in Gray W, McKee GT (eds): Diagnostic Cytopathology, ed 2. Hong Kong, Churchill-Livingstone, 2003, pp 492–503.

5 van Heerde P, Meyer CJLM, Noorduyn LA, van der Valk P: An Atlas and Textbook of Malignant Lymphomas. Cytology, Histopathology and Immunocytochemistry. London, Oxford University Press, 1996.

6 Orell S, Sterrett G, Whitaker D, van Heerde P, Miliasuskas J: Lymph nodes; in Orell S, Sterrett G, Whitaker D (eds): Fine Needle Aspiration Cytology, ed 5. London, Churchill-Livingstone, 2005, pp 83–125.

7 Melo JU, Catovsky D, Gregory WM, et al: The relationship between chronic lymphocytic leukemia and prolymphocytic leukemia. Br J Haematol 1987;65:23–29.

8 Lens O, De Schouwer PJ, Hamoudi RA, et al: p53 abnormalities in B-cell prolymphocytic leukemia. Blood 1997;89:2015–2023.

9 Isaacson PG, Piris MA, Catowsky D, et al: Splenic marginal zone lymphoma; in Jaffe ES, Harris NL, Stein H, Vardiman JW (eds): World Health Organization Classification of Tumors. Pathology and Genetics of Tumours of Haematopoietic and Lymphoid Tissue. Lyon, IARC Press, 2001, pp 135–137.

10 Thieblemont C, Felman P, Callet-Bauchu E, et al: Splenic marginal zone-lymphoma: a distinct clinical and pathological entity. Lancet Oncol 2003;4:95–103.

11 Chacon JI, Mollejo M, Munoz E, et al: Splenic marginal zone lymphoma: clinical characteristics and prognostic factors in a series of 60 patients. Blood 2002;100:1648–1654.

12 Matsushima AY, Hamele-Bena D, Osborne BM: Fine-needle aspiration biopsy findings in marginal zone B-cell lymphoma. Diagn Cytopathol 1999;20:190–198.

13 Frassoldati A, Lamparelli T, Federico M, et al: Hairy cell leukaemia: a clinical review based on 725 cases of the Italian Cooperative Group (ICGHCL) for hairy cell leukaemia. Leuk Lymphoma 1994;13:307–316.

14 Kaw YT, Artymyshyn RL, Schichman SA, et al: Recurrent hairy cell leukemia presenting as a large mesenteric mass diagnosed by fine needle aspiration cytology: a case report. Acta Cytol 1994;38:267–270.

15 Meara R, Reddy V, Arnoletti JP: Diagnosis of hairy cell leukemia by endoscopic ultrasound guided fine needle aspiration: a case report and review of recent literature. Cytojournal 2006; 3:1.

16 Grogan TM, Van Camp B, Kyle RA, et al: Plasma cell neoplasm; in Jaffe ES, Harris NL, Stein H, Vardiman JW (eds): World Health Organization Classification of Tumors. Pathology and Genetics of Tumours of Haematopoetic and Lymphoid Tissues. Lyon, IARC Press, 2001, pp 142–156.

17 Tani E, Santos GC, Svedmyr E, Skoog L: Fine-needle aspiration cytology and immunocytochemistry of soft-tissue extramedullary plasma-cell neoplasms. Diagn Cytopathol 1999;20:120–124.

18 Isaacson PG, Müller-Hermelink HK, Piris MA, et al: Extra nodal marginal zone B-cell lymphoma of mucosa-associated lymphoid tissue (MALT-lymphoma); in Jaffe ES, Harris NL, Stein H, Vardiman JW (eds): World Health Organization Classification of Tumors. Pathology and Genetics of Tumours of Haematopoietic and Lymphoid Tissue. Lyon, IARC Press, 2001, pp 157–160.

19 Isaacson PC, Nathwani BN, Piris MA, et al: Nodal marginal zone B-cell lymphoma; in Jaffe ES, Harris NL, Stein H, Vardiman JW (eds): World Health Organization Classification of Tumors. Pathology and Genetics of Tumours of Haematopoietic and Lymphoid Tissue. Lyon, IARC Press, 2001, p 161.

20 Crapanzano JP, Lin O: Cytologic findings of marginal zone lymphoma. Cancer. 2003;99: 301–309.

21 Murphy BA, Meda BA, Buss DH, Geisinger KR: Marginal zone and mantle cell lymphomas: assessment of cytomorphology in subtyping small B-cell lymphomas. Diagn Cytopathol 2003;28:126–130.

22 Kocjan G: Lymph nodes; in Kocjan G (ed): Clinical Cytopathology of the Head and Neck. London, Greenwich Medical Media, 2001.

23 Saikia UN, Dey P, Saikia B, Das A: Fine-needle aspiration biopsy in diagnosis of follicular lymphoma: cytomorphologic and immunohistochemical analysis. Diagn Cytopathol 2002; 26:251–256.

24 Rassidakis GZ, Tani E, Svedmyr E, Porwit A, Skoog L: Diagnosis and subclassification of follicle center and mantle cell lymphomas on fine-needle aspirates: a cytologic and immunocytochemical approach based on the Revised European-American Lymphoma (REAL) classification. Cancer 1999;87:216–223.

25 Sun W, Caraway NP, Zhang HZ, Khanna A, Payne LG, Katz RL: Grading follicular lymphoma on fine needle aspiration specimens: comparison with proliferative index by DNA image analysis and Ki-67 labeling index. Acta Cytol 2004;48:119–126.

26 Gagneten D, Hijazi YM, Jaffe ES, et al: Mantel cell lymphoma: a cytopathological and immunocytochemical study. Diagn Cytopathol 1996;14:32–37

27 Wojcik EM, Katz RL, Fanning TV, el-Naggar A, Ordonez NG, Johnston D: Diagnosis of mantle cell lymphoma on tissue acquired by fine needle aspiration in conjunction with immunocytochemistry and cytokinetic studies: possibilities and limitations. Acta Cytol 1995;39:909–915.

28 Bentz JS, Rowe LR, Anderson SR, Gupta PK, McGrath CM: Rapid detection of the t(11;14) translocation in mantle cell lymphoma by interphase fluorescence in situ hybridization on archival cytopathologic material. Cancer 2004;102:124–131.

29 Hughes JH, Caraway NP, Katz RL: Blastic variant of mantle-cell lymphoma: cytomorphologic, immunocytochemical, and molecular genetic features of tissue obtained by fine-needle aspiration biopsy. Diagn Cytopathol 1998;19:59–62.

30 Caraway N, Katz R: Lymph nodes; in Koss (ed): Diagnostic Cytology and Its Histopathologic Bases, ed 5. Philadelphia, Lippincott, 2006, pp 1186–1229.

31 Tani E, Johansson B, Skoog L: T-cell-rich B-cell lymphoma: fine-needle aspiration cytology and immunocytochemistry. Diagn Cytopathol 1998;18:1–4.

32 Tong TR, Lee KC, Chow TC, Chan OW, Lam WW, Lung R: T-cell/histiocyte-rich diffuse large B-cell lymphoma: report of a case diagnosed by fine needle aspiration biopsy with immunohistochemical and molecular pathologic correlation. Acta Cytol 2002;46: 893–898.

33 Shabb NS, Fahl M, Shabb B, et al: Fine needle aspiration of the mediastinum: a clinical, radiologic, cytologic and histologic study of 42 cases. Diagn Cytopathol 1998;19:428–436.

34 Hoda RS, Picklesimer L, Green KM, Self S: Fine needle aspiration of a primary mediastinal large B-cell lymphoma: a case report with cytologic histologic and flow cytometric considerations. Diagn Cytopath 2005;32:370–373.

35 Das DK, Gupta SK, Pathak IC, Sharma SC, Datta BN: Burkitt-type lymphoma. Diagnosis by fine needle aspiration cytology. Acta Cytol 1987;31:1–7.

36 Myong NH, Cho KJ, Choi SW, Jang JJ: Abdominal Burkitt's lymphoma diagnosed by fine needle aspiration cytology-a case report. J Korean Med Sci 1990;5:97–99.

37 Stastny JF, Almeida MM, Wakely PE Jr, Kornstein MJ, Frable WJ: Fine-needle aspiration biopsy and imprint cytology of small non-cleaved cell (Burkitt's) lymphoma. Diagn Cytopathol 1995;12:201–207.

38 Das DK, Sheikh ZA, Jassar AK, Jarallah MA: Burkitt- type lymphoma of the breast: diagnosis by fine-needle aspiration cytology. Diagn Cytopathol 2002;27:60–62.

39 Geramizadeh B, Kaboli R, Vasei M: Fine needle aspiration cytology of Burkitt's lymphoma presenting as a breast mass. Acta Cytol 2004; 48:285–286.

40 Jaffe ES and Wilson WH: Lymphoid granulomatosis; in Jaffe ES, Harris NL, Stein H, Vardiman JW (eds): World Health Organization Classification of Tumors. Pathology and Genetics of Tumours of Haematopoietic and Lymphoid Tissue. Lyon, IARC Press, 2001, pp 185–187.

41 Williams WL, Clark DA, Saiers JH: Fine needle aspiration diagnosis of lymphomatoid granulomatosis: a case report. Acta Cytol 1992; 36:91–94.

42 Vargas J, Arquelles M, Nevado M, et al: Fine needle aspiration biopsy of a cutaneous relapse of lymphomatoid granulomatosis: a case report. Acta Cytol 1993;37:205–208.

43 Kardos TF, Sprague RL, Wakely PE Jr, Frable WJ: Fine needle aspriation biopsy of lymphoblastic lymphoma and leukemia. AQ clinical, cytologic, and immunologic study. Cancer 1987;60:2448–2453.

44 Jacobs JC, Katz RL, Shabb N, el-Naggar A, Ordonez NG, Pugh W: Fine needle aspiration of lymphoblastic lymphoma: a multiparameter diagnostic approach. Acta Cytol 1992;36: 887–894.

45 Wakely PE Jr, Kornstein MJ: Aspiration cytopathology of lymphoblastic lymphoma and leukemia: the MCV experience. Pediatr Pathol Lab Med 1996;16:243–252.

46 Sah SP, Joshi A, Hanskak SG: Fine needle aspiration of precursor B lymphoblastic leukemia in an adult presenting as disseminated skin nodules. Acta Cytol 2005;49:399–450.

Chapter 5

T Cell Neoplasms

WHO Histological Classification of Mature T Cell and NK Cell Neoplasms

Leukemic/Disseminated
* T cell prolymphocytic leukemia
  T cell large granular lymphocytic leukemia
  Aggressive NK cell leukemia
* Adult T cell leukemia/lymphoma

Cutaneous
* Mycosis fungoides
* Sézary syndrome
* Primary cutaneous anaplastic large cell lymphoma

Other Extranodal
* Extranodal NK/T cell lymphoma, nasal type
  Enteropathy-type T cell lymphoma
  Hepatosplenic T cell lymphoma
  Subcutaneous panniculitis-like T cell lymphoma

Nodal
* Angioimmunoblastic T cell lymphoma
* Peripheral T cell lymphoma, unspecified
* Anaplastic large cell lymphoma

Neoplasm of Uncertain Lineage and Stage of Differentiation
  Blastic NK cell T-lymphoma
* Precursor T-lymphoblastic leukemia/lymphoma
(* Indicates subtypes described)

T Prolymphocytic Leukemia

Clinical Features

This rare subtype of leukemia is most often observed in old patients. In addition to lymphocytosis, lymph node involvement as well as infiltration of the skin and hepatosplenomegaly are frequently observed. Anemia and thrombocytopenia are common. T prolymphocytic leukemia (T-PLL) is highly aggressive and not curable with present therapy [1].

Cytology (fig. 5.1a)

The smear pattern is monomorphic of small- to medium-sized cells. The nuclei are mostly round but may in some cases show more nuclear irregularity and distinct nucleoli. Cases of PLL have a relatively abundant nongranular cytoplasm with frequent protrusions [2–4].

Differential diagnosis: B-CLL, mycosis fungoides (MF) and adult T cell lymphoma/leukemia.

Immunocytochemistry: The T-PLL cell is positive for T cell antigens (CD2, CD3, CD5 and CD7) (fig. 5.1b). CD4 is found in the majority of cases either without (2/3) or with (1/4) coexpression of CD8. Usually, a small (<5%) fraction of the cells is MIB-1 positive (fig. 5.1c).

Genetics: The T cell receptor is always rearranged. In addition, several abnormalities such as translocation (14;14), (8;8) and (X:14) have been reported.

Adult T Cell Lymphoma/Leukemia

Clinical Features
This subtype is caused by the human virus HTLV-1 and seen in adult patients with Japanese or Caribbean background (fig. 5.2a). Sporadic cases occur outside these areas. Chronic

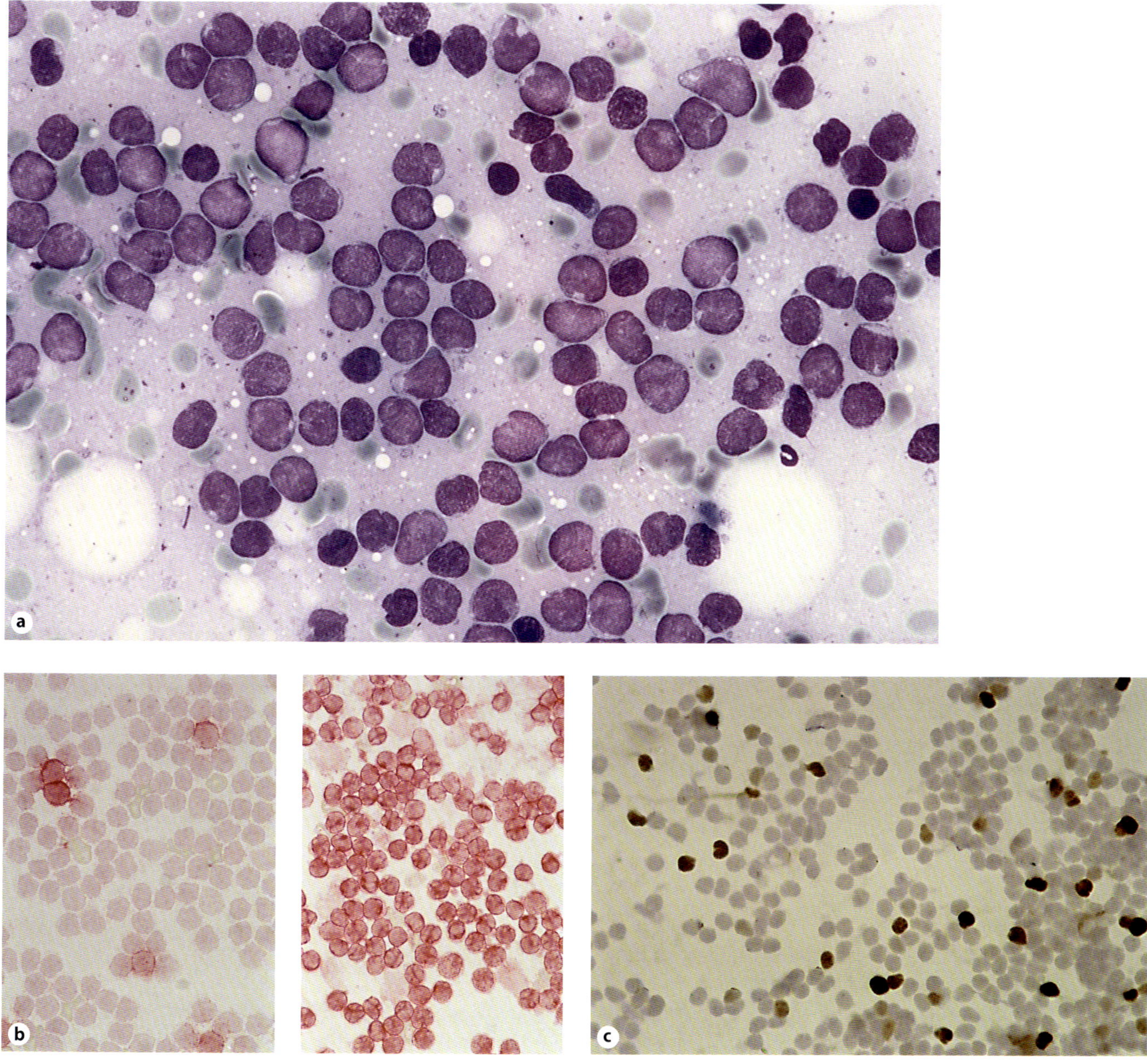

Fig. 5.1. a T-PLL. Smear showing monomorphic medium sized cells with irregular nuclei and sparse cytoplasm. (MGG, hpv). **b**. T-PLL. Immunocytochemistry on cytospin preparation shows a CD3+ tumor cell population (right) with few larger CD20+ cells (left). Alkaline phosphatase, high-power view. **c**. T-PLL. MIB-1 staining shows a low proliferation rate. Immunoperoxidase, high-power view.

and smoldering variants exist but the acute type is most common. Widespread lymphadenopathy, hepatosplenomegaly, papular skin lesions, leukemic blood picture and bone lesions with hypercalcemia dominate the clinical presentation [5].

Cytology (fig 5.2b)

There is a spectrum of lymphoid cells ranging in size from small to large, but medium-sized cells often dominate. The cells are polymorphic and have markedly irregular nuclei some with hyperlobation. The chromatin is coarse and nucleoli are distinct. There is a variable amount of cytoplasm staining from pale grey-blue to deep blue. Few cells will show cytoplasmic vacuoles [6, 7].

Differential diagnosis: Extreme variants of reactive lymphadenitis, diffuse large B cell lymphoma and lymphocyte depleted Hodgkin lymphoma.

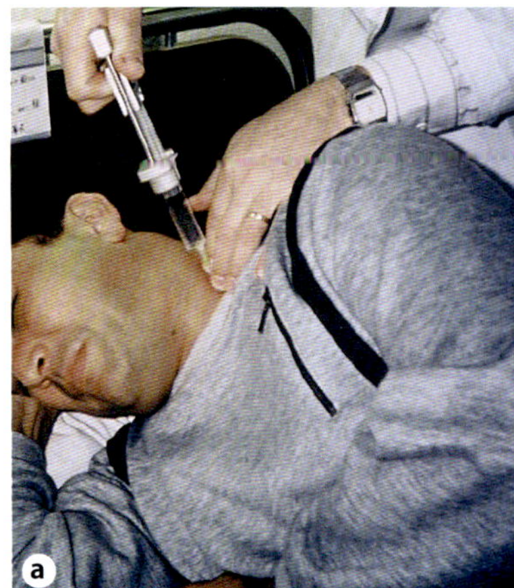
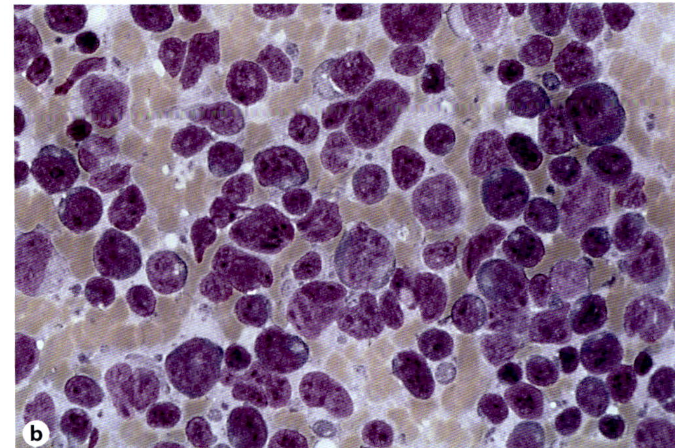
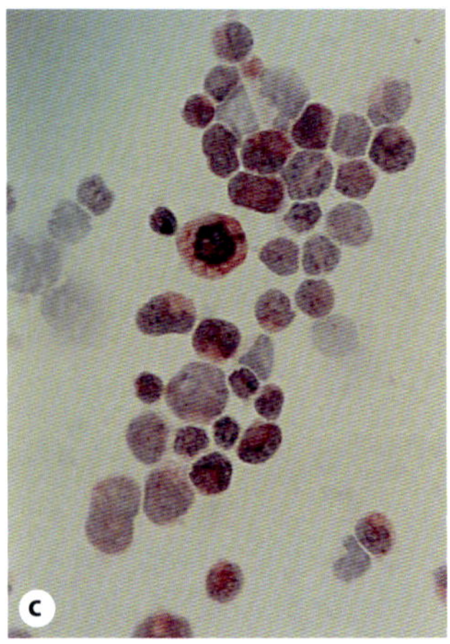
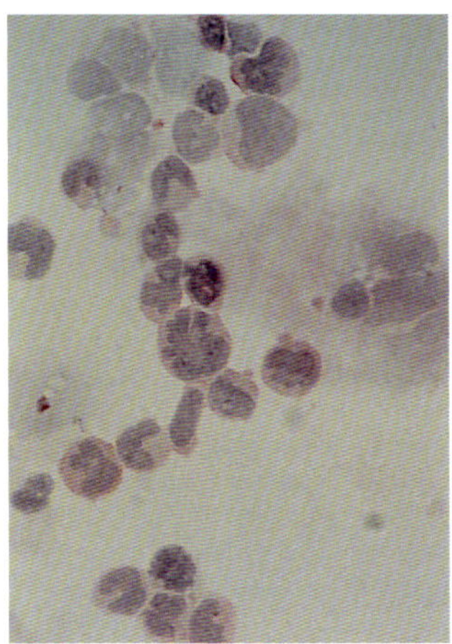

Fig. 5.2. a Aspiration from a cervical lymph node in a patient with adult T cell lymphoma HTLV-1+. **b** Adult T cell lymphoma. FNA smear with polymorphic immature tumor cells of varying size. The nuclei are irregular with prominent nucleoli and the cytoplasm deeply basophilic. MGG, high-power view. **c** Adult T cell lymphoma. Immunocytochemistry on cytospin preparation showing CD3 positivity (left) and weak positivity for CD4 (right). Alkaline phosphatase, high-power view.

Immunocytochemistry (fig. 5.2c): T cells antigens (CD2, CD3, CD4, CD5) are expressed along the entire spectrum of neoplastic cells. CD4 and CD25 are expressed in a majority of cases. The fraction of proliferating cells as measured by MIB-1 staining is high (over 50%).

Genetics: The T cell receptor genes are rearranged.

Mycosis Fungoides and Sezary Syndrome

Clinical Features (fig 5.3a)

Most patients are between 50 and 80 years of age. Both MF and Sezary syndrome (SS) show various forms of cutaneous involvement, e.g. erythrodermia. Plaques and palpable tumors are the presenting symptoms. Lymphadenopathy caused by tumor infiltrations is usually a late event. Extranodal manifestations such as soft tissue and CNS have been described. SS includes peripheral blood involvement. At present, no cure seems available, but local MF can have a protracted course while SS has a poor 5 years survival [8].

Cytology (fig. 5.3b)

The small tumor cell has an irregular 'folded' or cerebriform nucleus. The cytoplasm is sparse and blue in MGG. Large atypical cells can occasionally be detected. Late transformation to large T cell lymphoma is sometimes observed [2, 3, 8, 9].

Differential diagnosis: Dermatopathic lymphadenopathy and peripheral T cell lymphoma.

Immunophenotyping: The tumor cells express T cell antigens (CD2, 3, 4 and 5). A CD7 positivity is reported to be found in a minority of cases. The proliferative rate is low (<5%) as measured by MIB-1 staining.

Genetics: All cases have a clonal rearrangement of the T cell receptor. Several chromosomal alterations have been described but no specific changes seem to exist.

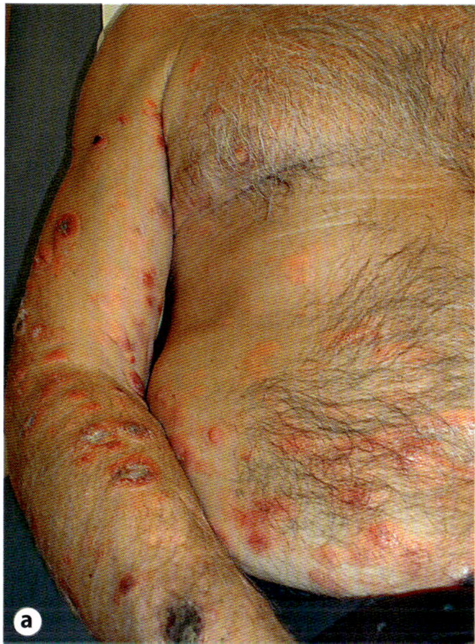

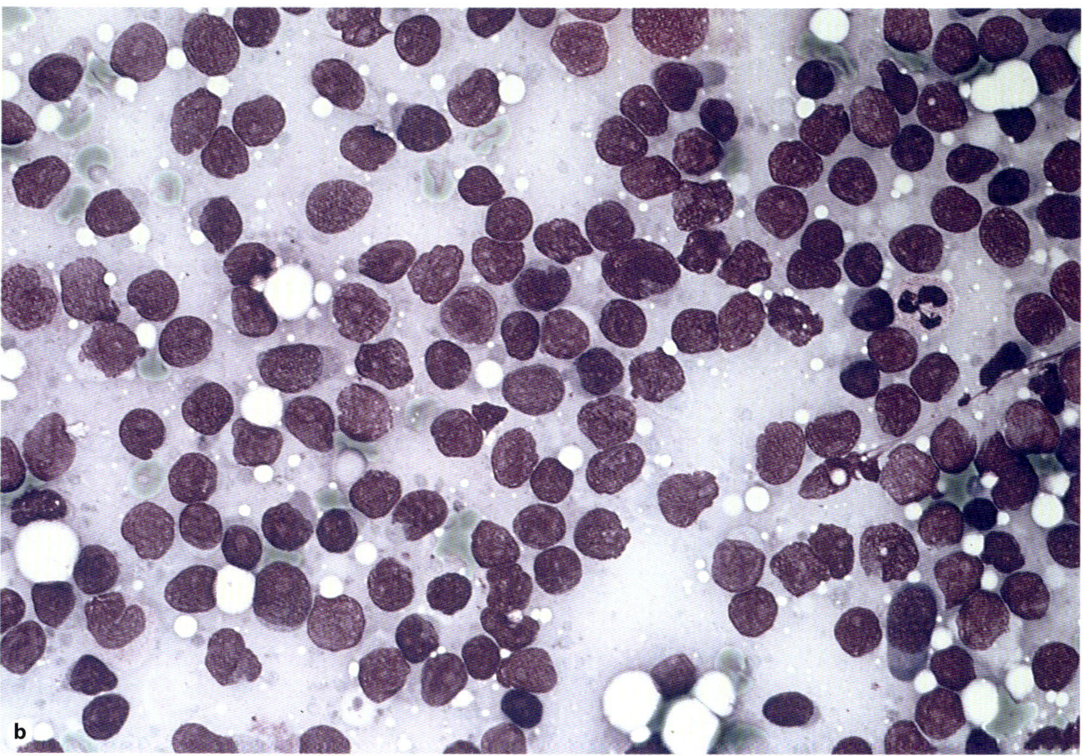

Fig. 5.3. a Mycosis fungoides. Cutaneous lesions. **b** Mycosis fungoides. Smear from aspirate shows small to medium sized lymphoid cells with irregular nuclei. MGG, high power view.

Extranodal NK/T Cell Lymphoma, Nasal Type

Clinical Features (fig. 5.4a)

This is a distinctly rare T cell lymphoma which is more prevalent in South America and Asia. It may affect children as well as adults. The paranasal sinuses are reported to be involved in the majority of cases, but other extranodal sites such as palate and skin are also commonly affected. Lymph nodes may be engaged in late stages. Radiotherapy or chemotherapy may induce complete remission [10].

Cytology (fig. 5.4b)

Smears are heterogeneous showing necrosis and many small and medium-sized atypical cells with irregular nuclei

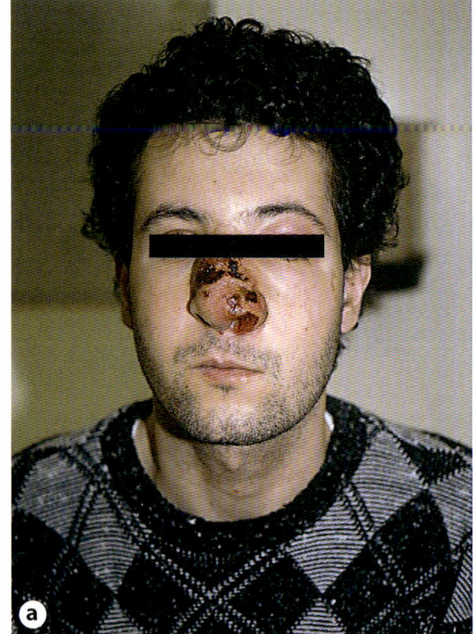
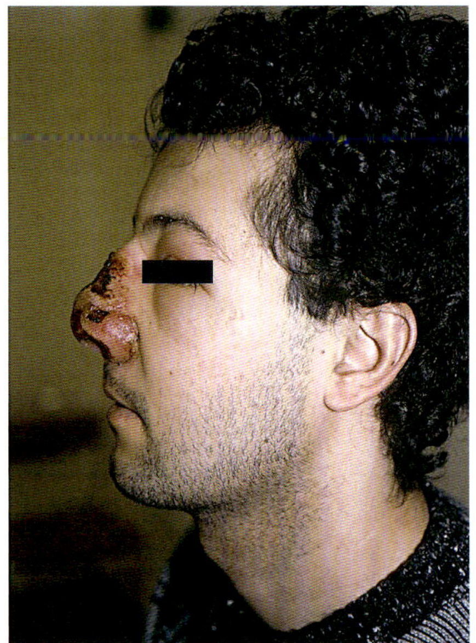

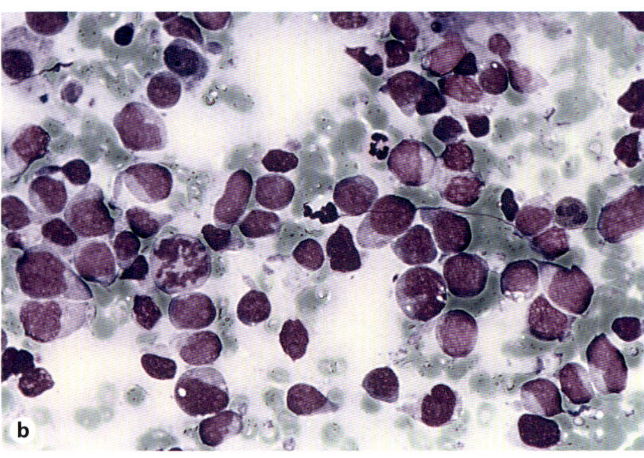

Fig. 5.4. a Extranodal NK/T cell lymphoma, nasal type. **b** Extranodal NK/T cell lymphoma, nasal type. Medium and large lymphatic cells, some with eccentric irregular nuclei. Mitoses are readily detected. MGG, high-power view.

and inconspicuous nucleoli. The pale cytoplasm is relatively abundant and may contain azurophilic granules. Mitotic figures are common. Large or anaplastic lymphoma cells can be found in varying numbers. There is often a rich admixture of eosinophils, plasma cells, benign mature lymphocytes and histiocytes [11].

Differential diagnosis: Other types of high-grade lymphomas.

Immunophenotype: The tumor cells express CD2 and CD56 while CD3, CD4 and CD5 are usually absent. EBV positivity can be demonstrated in a majority of the cases. The rate of cell proliferation is high.

Genetics: No specific translocation has been described. The T cell receptor genes are not rearranged.

Angioimmunoblastic T Cell Lymphoma

Clinical Features
The incidence peaks at around the age of 70 years and most patients have generalized disease at the time of diagnosis. Lymphadenopathy, fever, hepato- and splenomegaly, anemia and skin rash are common symptoms. Pleural effusion and ascites may also occur. Aggressive chemotherapy often induces remission which, however, may be of short duration, and the 5-year survival is less than 40% [12].

Cytology (fig. 5.5a,b)
Smears of aspirates present a complex cytomorphology. There is a mixture of small- to medium-sized lymphocytes with scanty pale cytoplasm, immunoblasts, eosinophils,

　　　T Cell Neoplasms

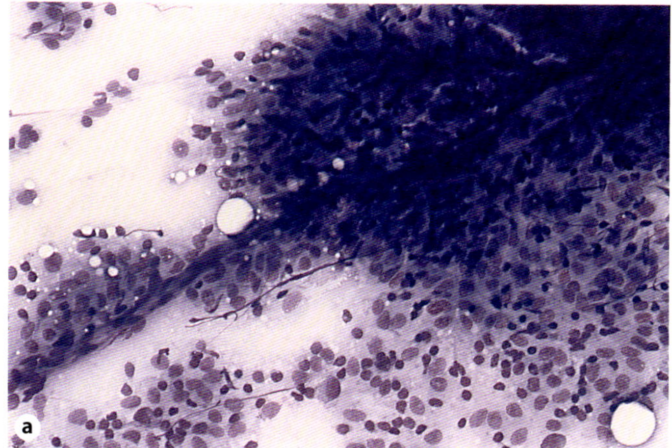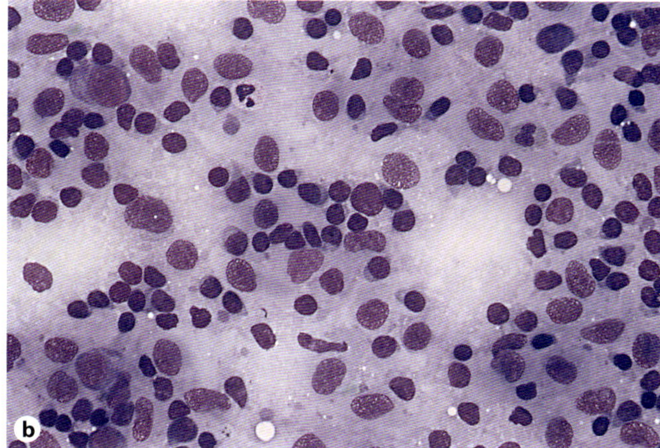

Fig. 5.5. a Angioimmunoblastic T cell lymphoma. The smear shows fragment of vessel with follicular dendritic cells extending from it and small to medium sized lymphoid cells without atypia. MGG, medium power view. **b** Angioimmunoblastic T cell lymphoma. Mixed population of cells with some intermediate-sized atypical cells with an irregular nuclei and poorly defined cytoplasm. In addition, some immunoblasts and eosinophils are seen. MGG, high-power view.

plasma cells and epitheloid histiocytes. The aspirate often contains fragments of thick vessels. The cytologic picture is seldom typical enough to allow a conclusive diagnosis of lymphoma. [2–4, 13, 4].

Differential diagnosis: Reactive hyperplasia, peripheral T cell lymphomas, adult T cell lymphoma/leukemia.

Immunophenotype: The tumor cells are CD3+ and there are usually CD4+ and CD8+ small cells.

Genetics: The T cell receptor genes are rearranged in a majority of the cases. Trisomy 3 or 5 is relatively common.

Peripheral T Cell Lymphoma, Unspecified

Clinical Features (fig 5.6a)

This is a rare subgroup in Western countries and is probably a mixture of disorders. The patients are usually adult and present with a variety of symptoms such as pruritus, lymphadenopathy, tumorous or diffuse infiltration of skin, liver, spleen and other viscera. In addition, bone marrow and peripheral blood are often involved. The clinical course is usually aggressive with a 5 years' survival of around 20% but occasional patients have long-lasting remissions after intense chemotherapy [15].

Cytology (fig. 5.6b–d)

The smear pattern is heterogeneous. The tumor cells are often medium to large in size and vary in shape. The nuclei are irregular, vary considerably in size and have distinct nucleoli. The cytoplasm is often abundant and stains pale grey-blue to dark blue in different cells from the same tumor. Mitoses are usually numerous. The complexity of the smear

is further enhanced by the admixture of eosinophils, plasma cells and epitheloid cells in varying proportions. Fragments of thin-walled vessels are often found. These rare tumors show such a broad variety of cells that it is difficult to describe their entire cytologic spectrum [2–4, 16–18].

Differential diagnosis: Reactive hyperplasia, other variants of T cell lymphoma in particular angioimmunoblastic T cell lymphoma and adult T cell lymphoma/leukemia.

Immunophenotyping (fig. 5.6e, f): A majority of the cases are CD4+ (T helper). The larger cells are often CD30+. Aberrant T cell antigen expression or deletion of pan-T antigens is highly suggestive of a neoplastic lymphoid population. These neoplasms are, however, difficult to diagnose conclusively using immunochemistry and TCR gene rearrangement analysis is often necessary to confirm the diagnosis. The proliferation rate is medium to high (30–70%) as analyzed by MIB-1 staining.

Genetics: The TCR genes are rearranged. In addition, there is a broad spectrum of alterations but no consistent abnormality.

Anaplastic Large Cell (CD30+) Lymphoma

Clinical Features

No age group is spared but young adults are overrepresented in this relatively rare entity. There are two major forms of the disease; one is cutaneous and the other systemic. The cutaneous form is seen mostly in adults and presents with skin tumors or nodules and may progress to involve other sites. The prognosis is good (90% 5-year survival) in pure cuta-

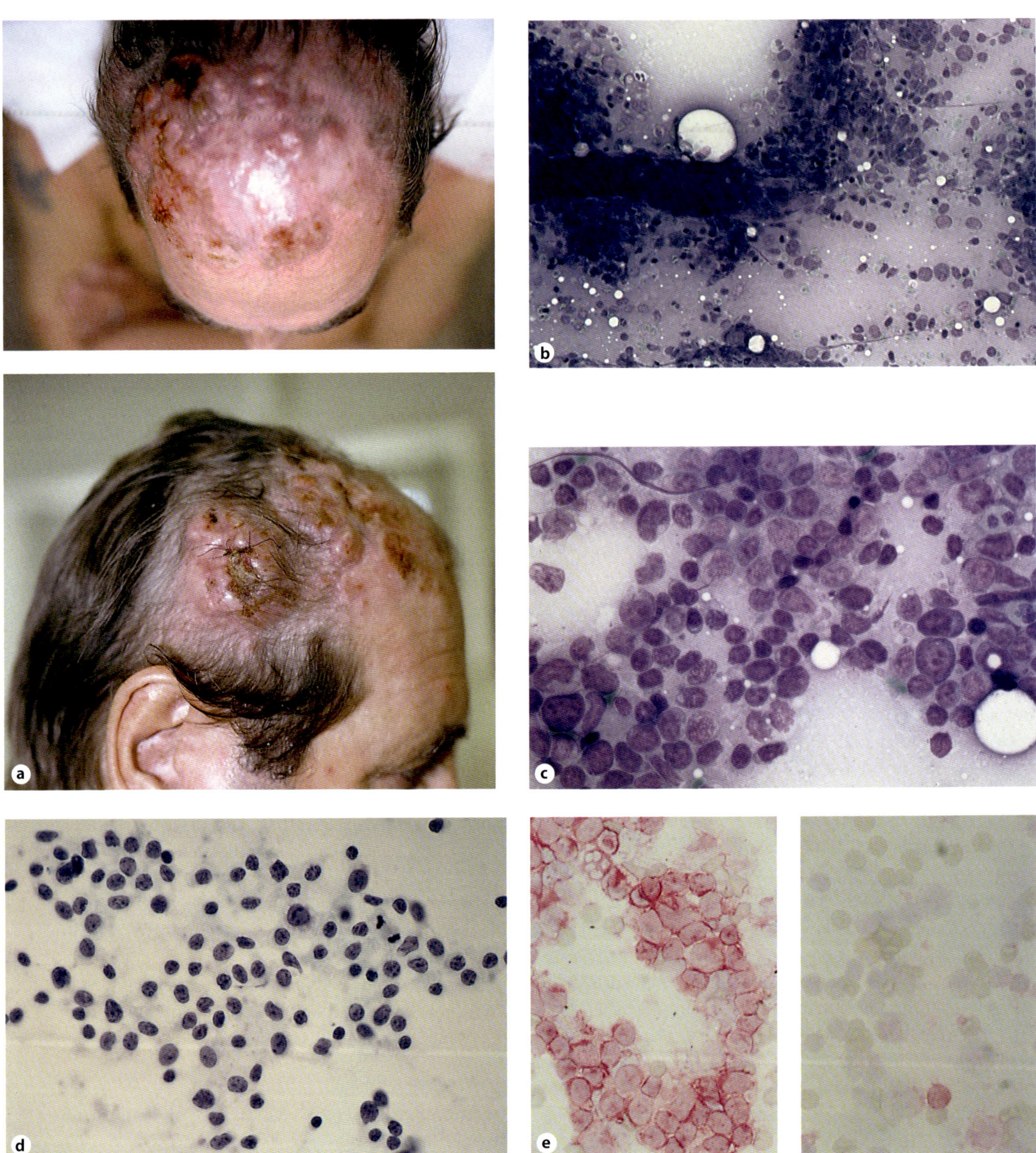

Fig. 5.6. a Peripheral T cell lymphoma involving the skin. **b** Peripheral T cell lymphoma. Smear shows a large fragment of a vessel and lymphoid cells of varying sizes with many large atypical cells. MGG, medium power view. **c** Peripheral T cell lymphoma. High power view of the case shown in **b**. MGG, high-power view. **d** Peripheral T cell lymphoma. Same aspirate shown in **b** stained with Papanicolaou. Medium and large cells with irregular nuclei with distinct nucleoli. One mitosis is seen. Pap, high-power view. **e** Peripheral T cell lymphoma. Immunocytochemistry on cytospin shows that the majority of the cells are positive for CD3 (left) and CD20+ cells are rarely found (right). Alkaline phosphatase, high-power view.

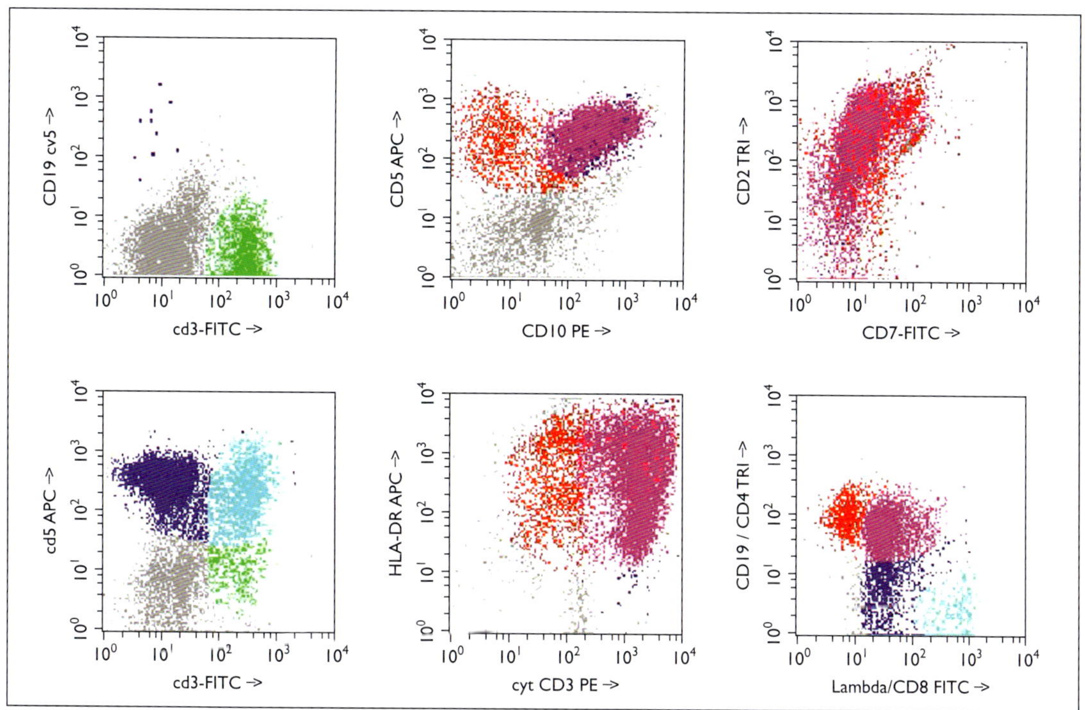

Fig. 5.6. f T cell lymphoma. Flow cytometry immunophenotyping of fine-needle aspirate from a lymph node with an angioimmunoblastic T cell lymphoma. Four-color flow cytometry was used. Upper left plot shows the presence of only few B cells (CD19+, blue dots), a population of CD3+ T cells (green dots) and a large population of cells negative for CD19 and CD3 (grey dots). Upper middle plot shows a large population of cells double positive for CD5 and CD10 (violet dots) and a smaller population of CD5+CD10− normal T cells. Upper right plot shows that most T cells were positive for CD2 and negative for CD7 (violet dots). A small population of normal T cells (CD2+/CD7+) was found. Lower left plot confirms that most CD5+ cells were negative for membrane CD3. Lower middle plot shows that most cells were positive for cytoplasmic CD3 and HLA-DR. Lower right plot shows that most T cells were stained positive for CD4 and weakly for CD8 (violet dots). Small populations of normal CD4+ T cells (red dots) and CD8+ T cells (cyan dots) are also present.

neous disease. The systemic type often presents with lymphadenopathy and extranodal (skin, bone, soft tissue and lung) infiltrates. Fever is a common symptom. Chemotherapy results in a high remission rate and the long-term survival is high for ALK positive tumors (5-year survival 80%) while ALK negative cases have a worse prognosis [19].

Cytology (fig. 5.7a, b)

The tumor cells of the cutaneous and systemic variants are similar. Two distinct variants have been described; a large cell and a small cell type. Smears from the more common large cell variant show large and polymorphic cells with a distinct pale grey-blue cytoplasm which is often vacuolated (fig. 5.7a). The nuclei vary considerably in size and shape and have several nucleoli. Typically horseshoe-shaped, ring formed and multilobated nuclei can be seen in most tumors of this subtype. Mitoses are frequent. In some cases, there is a rich admixture of granulocytes and macrophages [2, 3, 18, 20–30].

The small cell variant has medium-sized, less anaplastic tumor cells (fig. 5.7b). Cases with spindle cell forms have also been described.

Immunocytochemistry (fig. 5.7c–e): The tumor cells are typically CD30+, often EMA positive (systemic variant) as well as CD45. CD2 and CD4 positivity is found in a majority of the cases. The ALK protein is expressed in over 70% of the systemic cases and is typically absent in the primary cutaneous form. The positivity is cytoplasmic and nuclear but the expression can be restricted to one of these compartments (fig. 5.7d). A high proportion (>70%) of the tumors cells are MIB-1 positive (fig. 5.7e).

Genetics: The T cell receptor genes are rearranged in most cases. In addition, a translocation t(2;5) or t (1;2) is present in over 90% of the systemic cases.

Differential diagnosis: Other large anaplastic lymphomas, Hodgkin lymphoma of lymphocyte depletion type, metastasis from poorly differentiated carcinomas and melanomas.

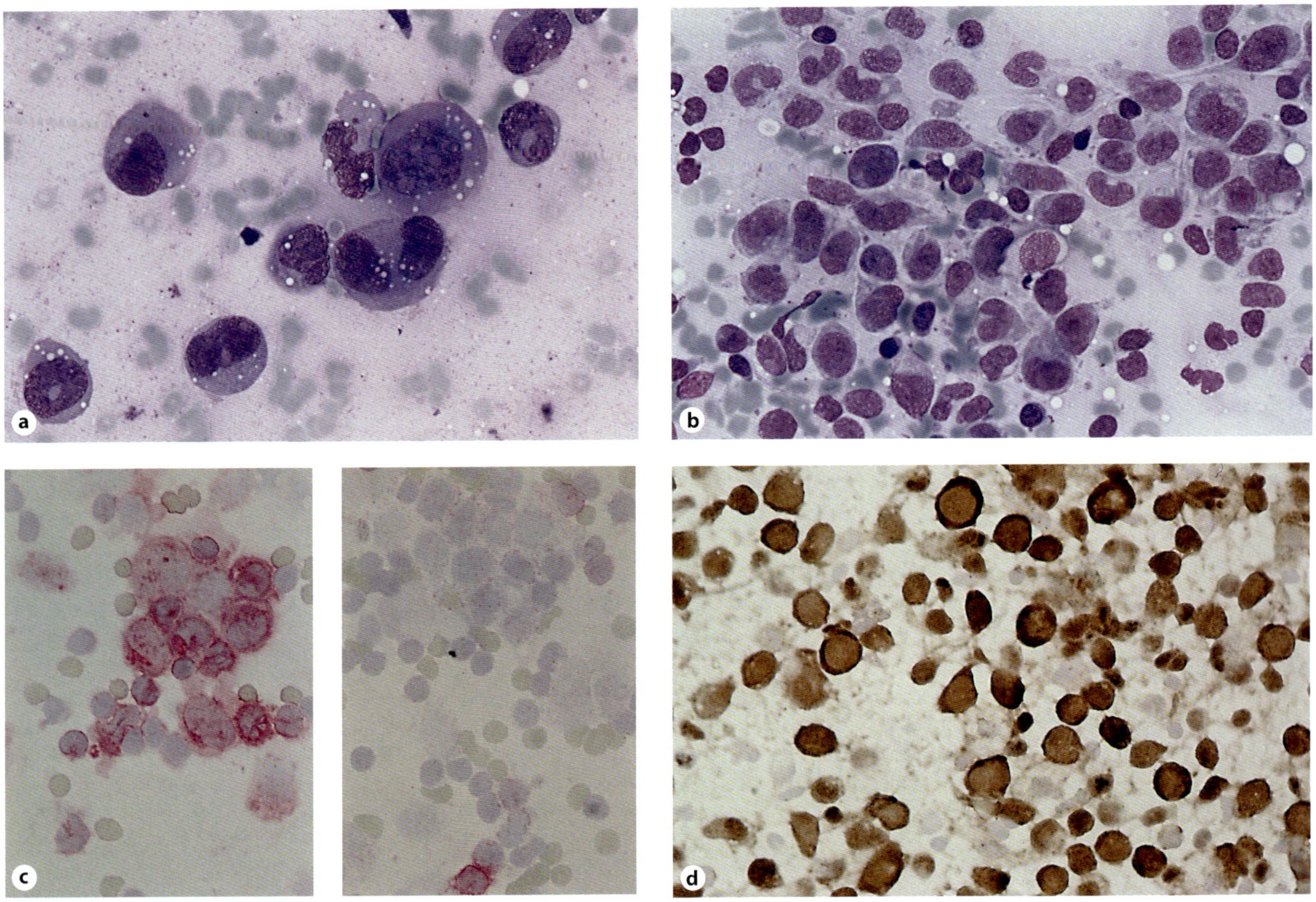

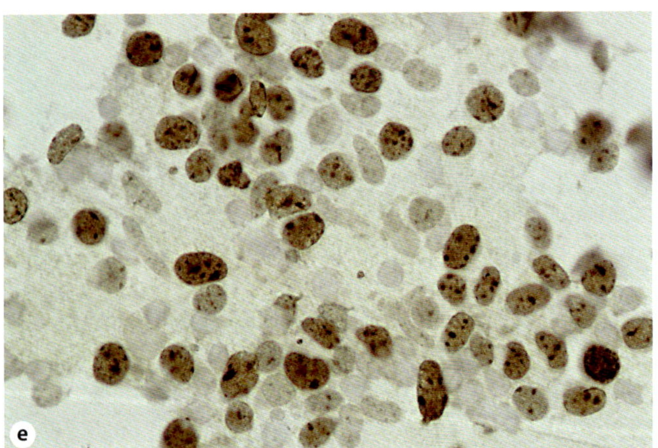

Fig. 5.7. a Anaplastic large cell lymphoma. Smear from a large cell variant shows polymorphic large cells with distinct blue-grey cytoplasm with vacuoles. Cells with ring-shaped nuclei and binucleated cells are represented. MGG, high-power view. b Anaplastic large cell lymphoma. Smear from a small cell type with kidney, horseshoe-shaped nuclei and some spindle-shaped cells. MGG, high-power view. c Anaplastic large cell lymphoma. Immunocytochemistry shows CD30 positivity in all tumor cells (left). CD3 is not expressed in the tumor cells (right). Alkaline phosphatase, high-power view. d Anaplastic large cell lymphoma. ALK-1 expression is visualized by brown nuclear and cytoplasmatic staining. Immunoperoxidase, high-power view. e A majority of the cells are proliferating as detected by MIB-1 staining. Immunoperoxidase, high-power view.

Precursor T Cell Leukemia/Lymphoma

Clinical Features

Most patients are young males, but children and adults can also be affected. A majority of the patients have bone marrow involvement but nodal and extranodal manifestations are common. Patients with high blast levels in the mar-row are classified as leukemic while a dominating mass disease is categorized as lymphoma. Bone marrow failure with anemia and infections is often the presenting symptom but some patients initially have a symptomatic space occupying mediastinal mass. If untreated the disease is highly aggressive and involvement of CNS, lymph nodes, skin and gonads occur. Chemotherapy will result in a high remission rate and a majority of these patients are cured.

　　　T Cell Neoplasms

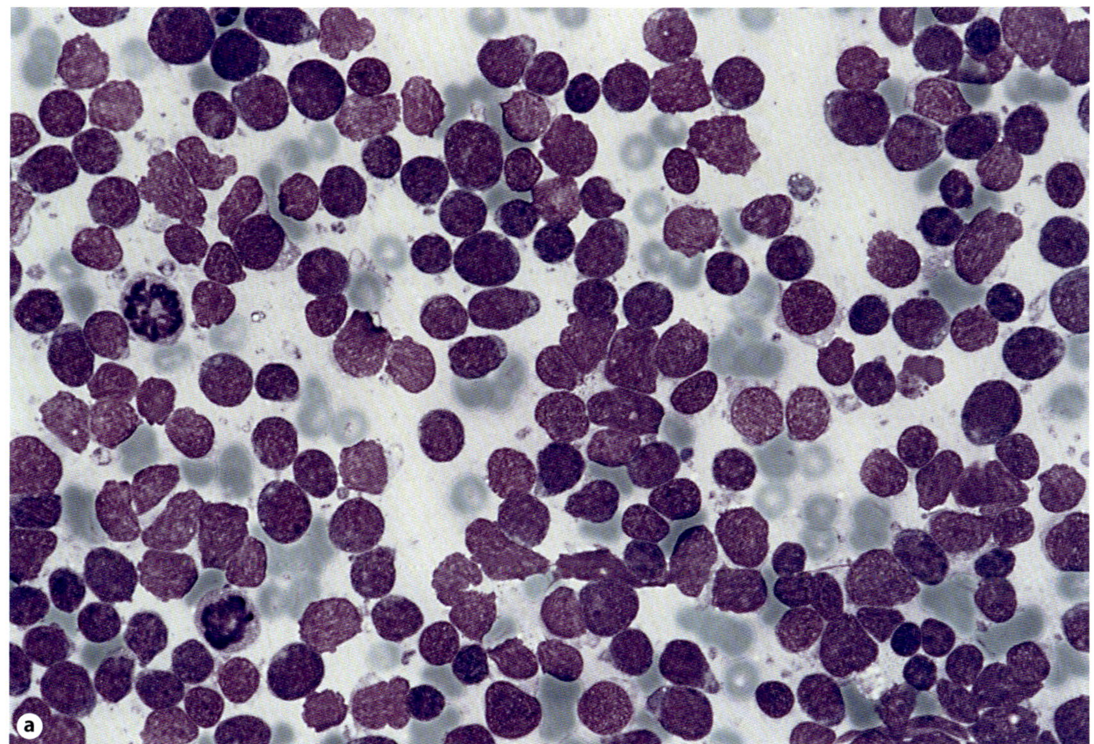

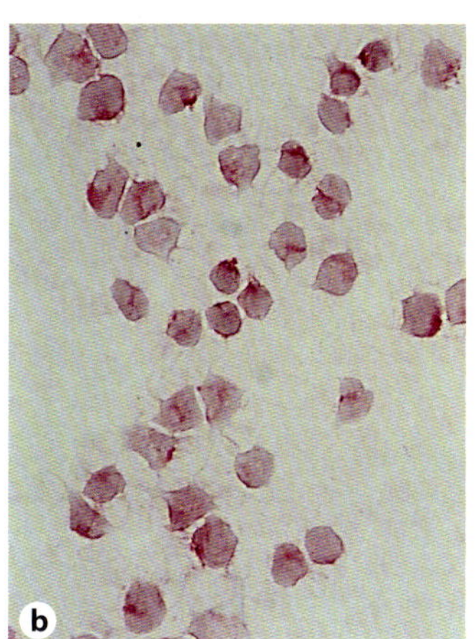

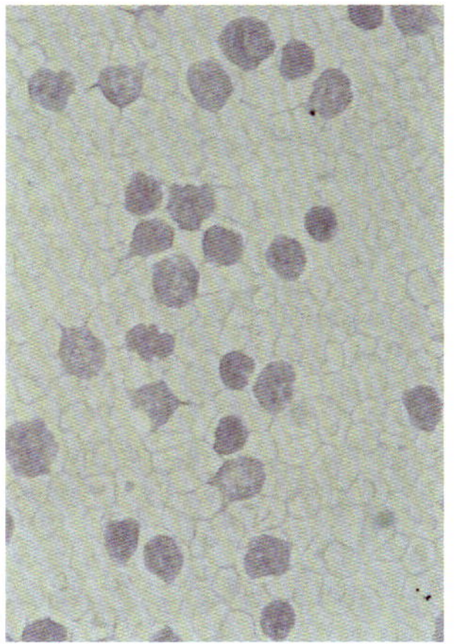

Fig. 5.8. a Precursor T cell ALL. Smear shows medium-sized blastic cells with sparse cytoplasm. Mitotic figures are frequent (MGG, high-power view). **b** Immunocytochemistry of the same aspirate as **a** shows that all cells are positive for CD3 (left) and negative for CD20 (right) (alkaline phosphatase, high-power view).

Cytology (fig. 5.8a)

Smears from aspirates show rounded mostly medium sized cell. The nuclei vary in shape and are often round to oval but convoluted forms also occur. The chromatin is even and nucleoli are rarely seen. The grey-blue cytoplasm is sparse and visible only in a limited part of the cell circumference. Usually, a few vacuoles can be found. Mitotic figures are common [2, 3, 18, 31–33].

Differential diagnosis: B-ALL, AML, Burkitt lymphoma.

Immunocytochemistry (fig. 5.8b): A majority of the cases express TdT, CD3 and CD7. CD4 and CD8 positivity is also common.

The proliferation rate is always higher than 50% as measured by MIB-1 staining.

Genetics: Rearrangement of the T cell receptor can be demonstrated in less than 50% of the cases.

References

1 Matutes E, Brito-Babapulle U, Swansbury et al: Clinical and laboratory features of 78 cases of T prolymphocytic leukaemia. Blood 1991;78:3269–3274.
2 Bizjak-Schwarzbartl M: Color Atlas of Non-Hodgkin's Lymphoma: Fine Needle Aspiration Biopsy. Ljubljana, Institute of Oncology, 1994.
3 Skoog L, Tani E: Lymph nodes; in Gray W, McKee GT (eds): Diagnostic Cytopathology, ed 2. Hong Kong, Churchill-Livingstone, 2003, pp 492–503.
4 Yao JL, Cangiarella JF, Cohen JM, Chhieng DC: Fine-needle aspiration biopsy of peripheral T-cell lymphomas: a cytologic and immunophenotypic study of 33 cases. Cancer 2001;93:151–159.
5 Shimoyama M: Diagnostic criteria and classification of clinical subtypes of adult T-cell leukaemia-lymphoma: a report from the Lymphoma Study Group. Br J Haematol 1991; 79:428–437.
6 Oshima K, Tani E, Masuda Y, Skoog L, Kikuchi M: Fine needle aspiration cytology of high grade T-cell lymphomas in human T-lymphotropic virus type 1 carriers. Cytopathology 1992;3:365–372.
7 Tong GX, Hernandez O, Yee HT, et al: Human T-lymphotropic virus type-1 related adult T-cell leukemia/lymphoma presenting as a parotid mass diagnosed by fine-needle aspiration biopsy. Diagn Cytopathol 2004;31:333–337.
8 Kim YH, Hoppe RT: Mycosis fungoides and the Sèzary syndrome. Semin Oncol 1999;26: 276–289.
9 Galindo LM, Garcia FU, Hanau CA, et al: Fine-needle aspiration biopsy in the evaluation of lymphadenopathy associated with cutaneous T-cell lymphoma (mycosis fungoides/Sezary syndrome). Am J Clin Pathol 2000;113: 865–871.
10 Chan JKC, Jaffe ES, Ralfkiaer E: Extranodal NK/T-cell lymphoma, nasal type; in Jaffe ES, Harris NL, Stein H, Vardiman JW (eds): World Health Organization Classification of Tumors. Pathology and Genetics of Tumours of Haematopoetic and Lymphoid Tissues. Lyon, IARC Press, 2001, pp 204–207.
11 Ng WK, Lee CY, Li AS, Cheung LK: Nodal presentation of nasal-type NK/T-cell lymphoma. Report of two cases with fine needle aspiration cytology findings. Acta Cytol 2003;47: 1063–1068.

12 Jaffe ES, Falfkiaer E: Angioimmunoblastic T-cell lymphoma; in Jaffe ES, Harris NL, Stein H, Vardiman JW (eds): World Health Organization Classification of Tumors. Pathology and Genetics of Tumours of Haematopoetic and Lymphoid Tissues. Lyon, IARC Press, 2001, pp 225–226.
13 Dey P, Radhika S, Das A: Fine-needle aspiration biopsy of angio-immunoblastic lymphadenopathy. Diagn Cytopathol 1996;15: 412–414.
14 Ng WK, Ip P, Choy C, Collins RJ: Cytologic findings of angioimmunoblastic T-cell lymphoma: analysis of 16 fine-needle aspirates over 9-year period. Cancer 2002;96: 166–173.
15 Ascari S, Zinzani Pl, Gherlinzoni F, et al: Peripheral T-cell lymphomas. Clinicopathologic study of 168 cases diagnosed according to the REAL classification. Ann Oncol 1997;8:583–592.
16 Tani E, Masuda Y, Skoog L, Ohshima K, et al: Cytology and immunocytochemistry of fine needle aspirates from peripheral T-cell lymphomas. Diagn Oncol 1991;1:133–139.
17 Al Shanqeety O, Mourad WA: Diagnosis of peripheral T-cell lymphoma by fine-needle aspiration biopsy: a cytomorphologic and immunophenotypic approach. Diagn Cytopathol 2000; 23:375–379.
18 Kocjan G: Lymph nodes; in Kocjan G (ed): Clinical Cytopathology of the Head and Neck. London, Greenwich Medical Media, 2001.
19 Anon: A clinical evaluation of the International Lymphoma Study Group classification of non-Hodgkin's lymphoma. The non-Hodgkin's Lymphoma Classification Project. Blood 1997; 89:3903–3918.
20 Brugieres L, Deley MC, Pacquement M, et al: CD30(+) anaplastic large-cell lymphoma in children: analysis of 82 patients enrolled in two consecutive studies of the French Society of Pediatric Oncology. Blood 1998;92: 3591–3598.
21 Tani E, Löwhagen T, Nasiell K, et al: Fine needle aspiration cytology and immunocytochemistry of large cell lymphomas expressing the Ki-1 antigen. Acta Cytol 1989;33:359–362.
22 Dusenbery D, Jones DB, Sapp KW, et al: Cytologic findings in the sarcomatoid variant of large cell anaplastic (Ki-1) lymphoma: a case report. Acta Cytol 1993;37:508–514.

23 McCluggage WG, Anderson N, Herron B, et al: Fine needle aspiration cytology, histology and immunohistochemistry of anaplastic large cell Ki-1-positive lymphoma: a report of three cases. Acta Cytol 1996;40:779–785.
24 Bizjak-Schwarzbartl M: Large cell anaplastic Ki-1+ non-Hodgkin's lymphoma vs. Hodgkin's disease in fine needle aspiration biopsy samples. Acta Cytol 1997;41:351–356.
25 Jayaram G, Abdul Rahman N: Cytology of Ki-1 positive anaplastic large cell lymphoma: a report of two cases. Acta Cytol 1997;41(suppl 4):1253–1260.
26 Gatter KM, Rader A, Braziel RM: Fine-needle aspiration biopsy of anaplastic large cell lymphoma, small cell variant with prominent plasmacytoid features: case report. Diagn Cytopathol 2002;26:113–116.
27 Mourad WA, al Nazer M, Tulbah A: Cytomorphologic differentiation of Hodgkin's lymphoma and Ki-1+ anaplastic large cell lymphoma in fine needle aspirates. Acta Cytol 2003;47:744–748.
28 Ng WK, Ip P, Choy C, Collins RJ: Cytologic and immunocytochemical findings of anaplastic large cell lymphoma: analysis of ten fine-needle aspiration specimens over a 9-year period. Cancer 2003;99:33–43.
29 Kim SE, Kim SH, Lim BJ, et al: Fine needle aspiration cytology of small cell variant of anaplastic large cell lymphoma: a case report. Acta Cytol 2004;48:254–258.
30 Tamiolakis D, Georgiou G, Prassopoulos P, et al: Neutrophil-rich anaplastic large cell lymphoma (NR-ALCL) mimicking lymphadenitis: a study by fine-needle aspiration biopsy. Leuk Lymphoma 2004;45:1309–1310.
31 Tani E, Maeda S, Fröstad B, et al: Aspiration cytology with phenotyping and clinical presentation of childhood lymphomas Diagn Oncol 1993;3:294–301.
32 Jacobs JC, Katz RL, Shabb N, el-Naggar A: Fine needle aspiration of lymphoblastic lymphoma: a multiparameter diagnostic approach. Acta Cytol 1992;36:887–894.
33 Wakely PE Jr, Kornstein MJ: Aspiration cytopathology of lymphoblastic lymphoma and leukemia: the MCV experience. Pediatr Pathol Lab Med 1996;16:243–257.

T Cell Neoplasms

Chapter 6

Hodgkin Lymphoma

WHO Histological Classification, Hodgkin Lymphoma

Classic Hodgkin Lymphoma
* Nodular sclerosis
* Mixed cellularity
* Lymphocyte rich
* Lymphocyte depleted
* *Nodular lymphocyte predominant Hodgkin*
(* Indicates subtypes described)

Hodgkin lymphoma is today divided in two distinct groups: classical Hodgkin lymphoma, and nodular lymphocyte-predominant Hodgkin lymphoma [1]. The classical type includes 4 subtypes: (1) nodular sclerosis, (2) mixed cellularity, (3) lymphocyte rich, and (4) lymphocyte depleted. All these subtypes have mononuclear (Hodgkin) and multinucleated (Reed-Sternberg) cells with identical phenotype as well as genetic features. However, their clinical and cytologic features differ and they will therefore be described separately. It should be pointed though out that subtyping of classical Hodgkin lymphoma has little prognostic information compared with the clinical stage [2].

Nodular lymphocyte-predominant Hodgkin lymphoma differs from classical Hodgkin lymphoma with respect to clinical behavior, cytomorphology and immunocytophenotype and will thus be discussed separately [1].

Classical Hodgkin Lymphoma

(1) Nodular Sclerosis Variant

Clinical Features (fig. 6.1a)
Young adults dominate and children are rarely affected. Mediastinal and cervical lymph nodes are almost always involved. Spleen, lung and bone marrow involvement is seen in less than 10% of the patients. The dominating symptom is lymphadenopathy but fever, weight loss and night sweats are also common. Modern radio- and chemotherapy results in a high cure rate [1, 2].

Cytologic Features (fig. 6.1b, c)
The smears are often scanty due to the sclerosis and therefore several nodes in the same area should be sampled if possible (fig. 6.1b). In general, smaller nodes give more cellular smears with more tumor cells. The smears are dominated by small mature lymphoid cells. The tumor cells may be rare and careful search is often needed to identify them. The Hodgkin cell has a large nucleus with a distinct nucleolus and a large pale blue cytoplasm. The Reed-Sternberg cell usually has a bilobated nucleus with distinct nucleoli. Occasionally, the nucleus is multilobated. The cytoplasm is abundant and poorly outlined (fig. 6.1c). Collagen fragments and fibroblasts as well as eosinophilic granulocytes are common [3–14].

Differential diagnosis: See below.

Immunocytochemistry (fig. 6.1d): The tumor cells express CD30 and may be CD15 positive. Weak positivity for CD20 can be seen in some cases. Expression of CD45 and EMA is never seen. It should be noted that Hodgkin and Reed-Sternberg cells often lose their cytoplasm in cytospin preparations. CD30 positivity is therefore often weak in contrast to that seen in anaplastic large cell lymphoma of the Ki-1 type. A majority of the tumor cells are proliferating as measured by MIB-1 staining.

(2) Mixed Cellularity Variant

Clinical Features
This subtype accounts for approximately 1/5 of Hodgkin cases and is most frequent in middle-aged men. An

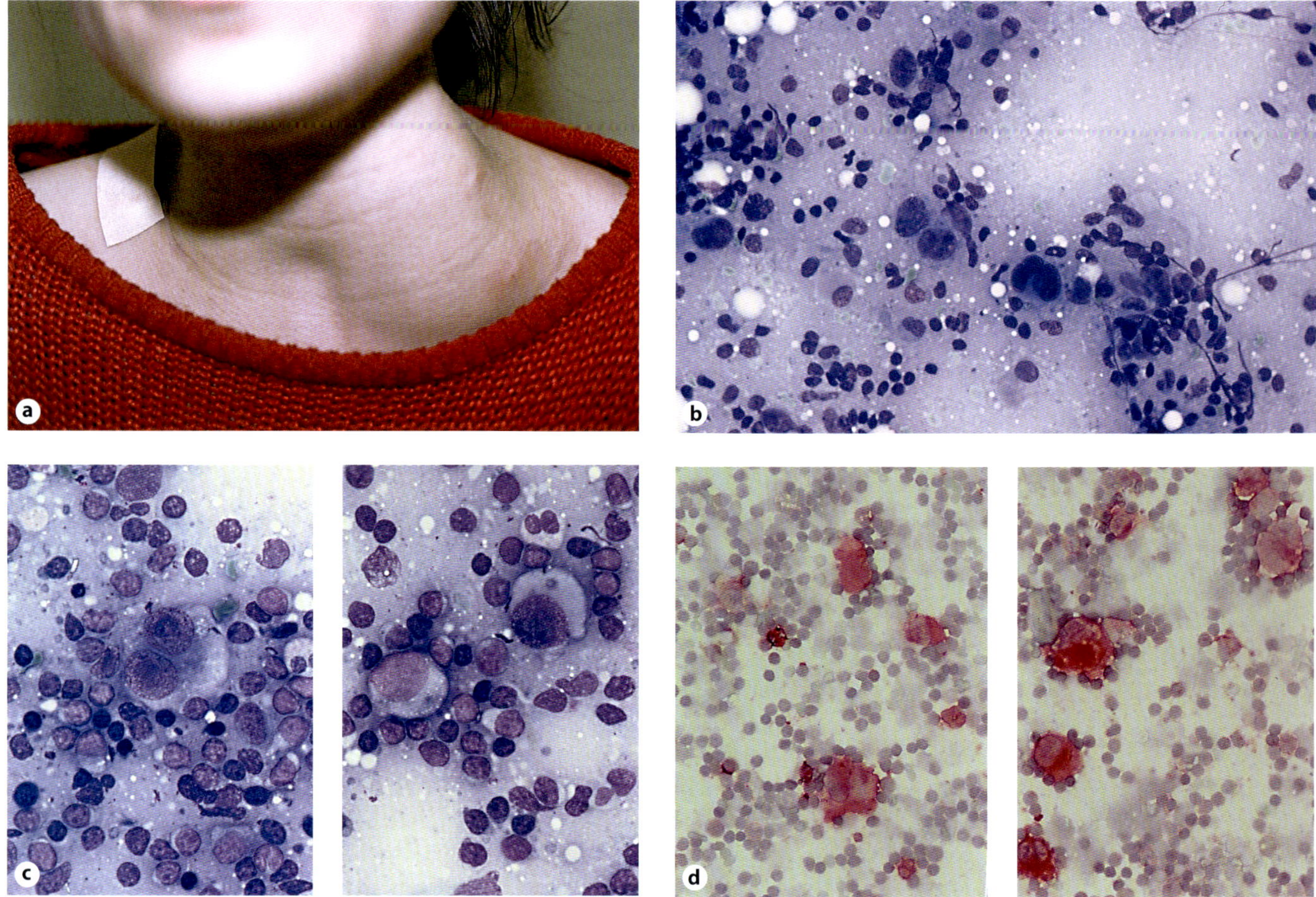

Fig. 6.1. a Hodgkin lymphoma. Typical clinical presentation with firm lymph nodes in the neck in a young patient. **b** Hodgkin lymphoma, nodular sclerosis variant. Sparse smear with mature lymphocytes and large Hodgkin cells and some binucleated cells of Reed-Sternberg type. MGG, medium-power view. **c** Hodgkin lymphoma. Binucleated Reed-Sternberg cell (left) with prominent nucleoli and two mononucleated Hodgkin cells (right) with distinct cytoplasm and large nucleolus. MGG, high-power view. **d**. Hodgkin lymphoma. Immunocytochemistry shows tumor cells positive for CD30 (right) and CD15 (left). Alkaline phosphatase, medium-power view.

association with HIV infection has been described. Generalized lymphadenopathy is common as well as weight loss and fever. The survival rate is similar to that of the other subtypes [1, 2].

Cytologic Features (fig. 6.2)
The Hodgkin and Reed-Sternberg cells are similar to those found in the nodular sclerosis variant. However the background cell population is different. The lymphocytes are often of small to medium in size but the centroblast may also be seen. Eosinophils, neutrophils and plasma cells are often present. In addition, histiocytes with an epitheloid differentiation are common. In rare cases, granulocytes dominate and the cytology may mimic that of suppurative lymphadenitis [3, 5, 7–9, 15–17].
Differential diagnosis: See below.

Immunocytochemistry: The tumor cells have the same phenotype as that of nodular sclerosis. However, LMP1 expression is found in a majority of cases.

(3) Lymphocyte-Rich Variant

Clinical Features
This rare subtype is most often found in middle-aged to elderly patients. Peripheral lymph node adenopathy is common but widely disseminated disease is uncommon. The prognosis is good [1, 2].

Cytologic Features (fig. 6.3)
The tumor cells are rare but identical to Hodgkin and Reed-Sternberg cells of the other subtypes. The background

Hodgkin Lymphoma

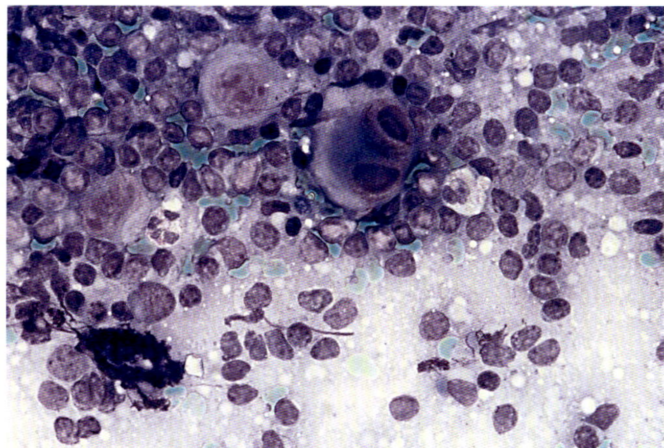

Fig. 6.2. Hodgkin lymphoma, mixed cellularity variant. Smear shows mononuclear tumor cells and a Reed-Sternberg binucleated cell with huge nucleoli in a background dominated by small lymphocytes and few eosinophils. MGG, high-power view.

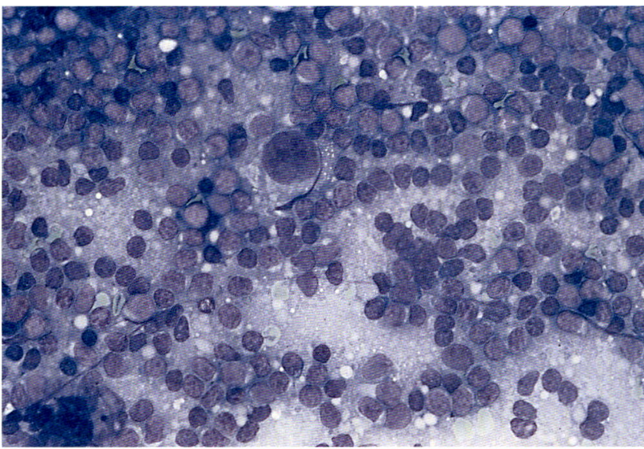

Fig. 6.3. Hodgkin lymphoma, lymphocyte-rich variant. Smear shows small reactive lymphocytes and one large tumor cell of Hodgkin type. MGG, high-power view.

is dominated by a full spectrum of lymphoid cells ranging from small mature cells to germinal cells. Eosinophils and histiocytes are not present [3, 5, 7–9].

Differential diagnosis: See below.

Immunocytochemistry: Identical to that of the other subtypes.

(4) Lymphocyte-Depleted Variant

Clinical Features

This is a rare subtype which is mostly seen in middle-aged men and then often in association with HIV infection. Deep lymph nodes and bone marrow are often engaged. Most patients present with weight loss and fever. The clinical course is comparable to the other subtypes, but in HIV-infected patients the disease is aggressive.

Cytologic Features (fig. 6.4)

Hodgkin and Reed-Sternberg cells with typical cytologic features dominate the smears. Small- to medium-sized lymphoid cells are always present [3, 5, 7–9, 18].

Differential diagnosis: T cell-rich B cell lymphoma (monoclonal, B phenotype), anaplastic large cell lymphoma of Ki-1 type (CD30, CD45, EMA, ALK, T cell phenotype) and nodular lymphocyte predominant Hodgkin lymphoma (CD20, CD45, monoclonal). Metastatic carcinoma (CK, EMA) or melanoma (S-100, HMB45).

Immunocytochemistry: The immunophenotype of the tumor cells is identical to that of the other subtypes.

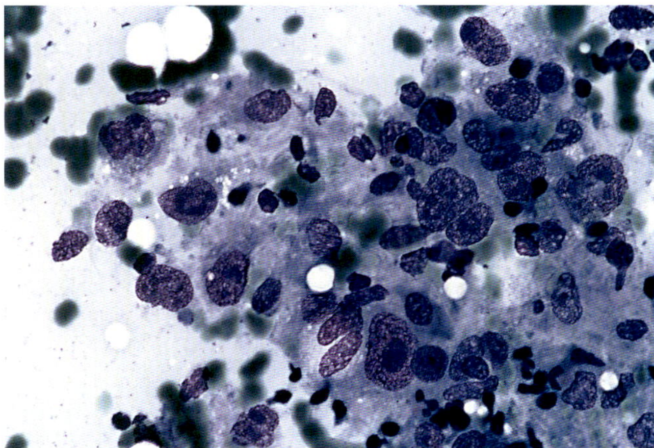

Fig. 6.4. Hodgkin lymphoma, lymphocyte depleted variant. Several large tumor cells are seen. MGG, high-power view.

Nodular Lymphocyte Predominant Hodgkin Lymphoma

Clinical Features

This lymphoma is most frequent in middle-aged patients. Peripheral lymphadenopathy, often localized, is the common presenting symptom. A high responsive rate is common and most patients are cured [19]. Transformation to large B cell lymphoma has, however, been reported [20].

Cytologic Features (fig. 6.5a, b)

The large tumor cells are often sparse and can be difficult to identify in the highly cellular background of small-to-large

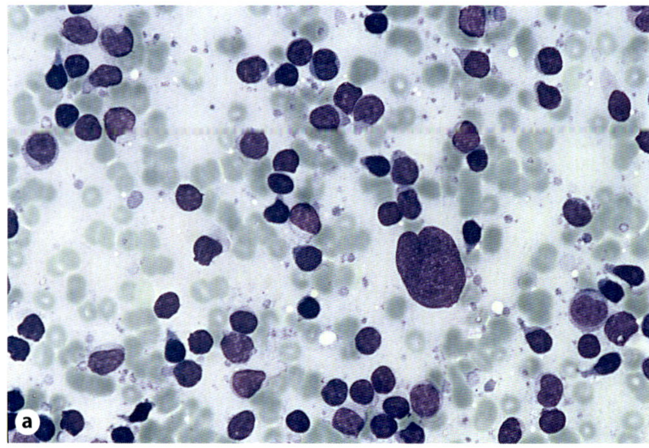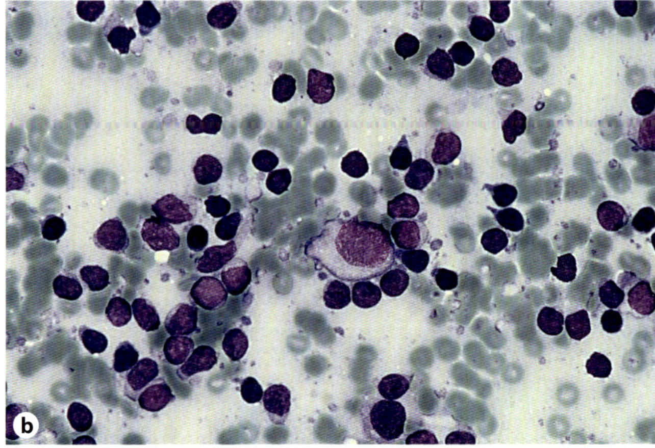

Fig. 6.5. Hodgkin lymphoma, nodular lymphocyte predominant type. A large naked folded tumor cell nucleus with small nucleoli and many reactive lymphocytes (**a**) and a large tumor cell with distinct cytoplasm (**b**). MGG, high-power view.

type lymphocytes. The tumor cell can either have a folded or multilobated nucleus with relatively small nucleoli or a round nucleus with a distinct nucleolus. Histiocytes and plasma cells are frequently observed. The paucity of tumor cells makes the cytologic diagnosis challenging.

Differential diagnosis: T cell-rich B cell lymphoma (has similar phenotype and is cytologically similar), Hodgkin lymphoma lymphocyte-rich (CD30, CD15), diffuse large B cell lymphoma (similar phenotype but the tumor cells are usually numerous).

Immunocytochemistry: The tumor cell is CD20, CD45, CD79a, Oct2 positive and most cases express monoclonal light chains. CD15 and CD30 are not expressed.

References

1 Stein H, Delsol G, Pileri S, et al: Hodgkin lymphomas; in Jaffe ES, Harris NL, Stein H, Vardiman JW (ed): World Health Organization Classification of Tumors. Pathology and Genetics of Tumours of Haematopoetic and Lymphoid Tissues. Lyon, IARC Press, 2001, pp 240–253.

2 Specht L, Hasenclever D: Prognostic factors of Hodgkin's disease; in Mauch P, Armitage JO, Diehl V (eds): Hodgkin's Disease. Philadelphia, Lippincott/Williams & Wilkins, 1999, p 295.

3 Skoog L, Tani E: Lymph nodes; in Gray W, McKee GT (eds): Diagnostic Cytopathology, ed 2. Hong Kong, Churchill-Livingstone, 2003, pp 492–503.

4 Orell S, Sterrett G, Walters M, Whitaker D, van Heerde P: Lymph nodes; in Orell S, Sterrett G, Walters M, Whitaker D (eds): Fine Needle Aspiration Cytology, ed 4. London, Churchill-Livingstone, 2005, pp 101–105.

5 Das D: Lymph nodes; in Bibbo M (ed): Comprehensive Cytopathology. 2nd ed. Philadelphia. W.B. Saunders Company; 1997, pp 703–731.

6 Kocjan G: Lymph nodes; in Kocjan G (ed): Clinical Cytopathology of the Head and Neck. London, Greenwich Medical Media, 2001.

7 Moriarty AT, Banks ER, Bloch T: Cytologic criteria for subclassification of Hodgkin's disease using fine-needle aspiration. Diagn Cytopathol 1989;5:122–125.

8 Das DK, Gupta SK: Fine needle aspiration cytodiagnosis of Hodgkin's disease and its subtypes. II. Subtyping by differential cell counts. Acta Cytol 1990;34:337–341.

9 Das DK, Gupta SK, Datta BN, Sharma SC: Fine needle aspiration cytodiagnosis of Hodgkin's disease and its subtypes. I. Scope and limitations. Acta Cytol 1990;34:329–336.

10 Tani E, Maeda S, Fröstad B, Björk O, Löwhagen T, Skoog L: Aspiration cytology with phenotyping and clinical presentation of childhood lymphomas. Diagn Oncol 1993;3:294–301.

11 Fulciniti F, Vetrani A, Zeppa P, Giordano G, Marino M, De Rosa G, Palombini L: Hodgkin's disease: diagnostic accuracy of fine needle aspiration; a report based on 62 consecutive cases. Cytopathology 1994;5:226–233.

12 Jimenez-Heffernan JA, Vicandi B, Lopez-Ferrer P, Hardisson D, Viguer JM: Value of fine needle aspiration cytology in the initial diagnosis of Hodgkin's disease: analysis of 188 cases with an emphasis on diagnostic pitfalls. Acta Cytol 2001;45:300–306.

13 Chieng DC, Cangiarella JF, Symmans WF, Cohen JM: Fine-needle aspiration cytology of Hodgkin disease: a study of 89 cases with emphasis on false-negative cases. Cancer 2001; 93:52–59.

14 Moreland WS, Geisinger KR: Utility and outcomes of fine-needle aspiration biopsy in Hodgkin's disease. Diagn Cytopathol 2002; 26:278–282.

15 Fulciniti F, Zeppa P, Vetrani A, Troncone G, Palombini L: Hodgkin's disease mimicking suppurative lymphadenitis: a possible pitfall in fine-needle aspiration biopsy cytology. Diagn Cytopathol 1989;5:282–285.

16 Tani E, Ersoz C, Svedmyr E, Skoog L: Fine-needle aspiration cytology and immunocytochemistry of Hodgkin's disease, suppurative type. Diagn Cytopathol 1998;18:437–440.

17 Vicandi B, Jimenez-Heffernan JA, Lopez-Ferrer P, Gamallo C, Viguer JM: Hodgkin's disease mimicking suppurative lymphadenitis: a fine-needle aspiration report of five cases. Diagn Cytopathol 1999;20:302–306.

18 Grosso LE, Collins BT, Dunphy CH, Ramos RR: Lymphocyte-depleted Hodgkin's disease: diagnostic challenges by fine-needle aspiration. Diagn Cytopathol 1998;19:66–69.

19 Diehl V, Franklin J, Sextro M, et al: Clinical presentation and treatment of lymphocyte predominance Hodgkin's disease; in Mauch P, Armitage JO, Diehl V (eds): Hodgkin's Disease. Philadelphia, Lippincott/Williams & Wilkins, 1999, p 563.

20 Hansmann ML, Stein H, Fellbaum C, Hui PK, Parwaresch MR, Lennert K: Nodular paragranuloma can transform into high-grade malignant lymphoma of B type. Hum Pathol 1989;20: 1169–1175.

Immunodeficiency-Associated Lymphoproliferative Disorders

WHO Histological Classification of Immunodeficiency-Associated Lymphoproliferative Disorders

* Human immunodeficiency virus-related lymphomas
* Post-transplant lymphoproliferative disorder, polymorphic
(* Indicates subtypes described)

Lymphadenopathy in HIV-Infected Patients

(1) Hyperplasia
(2) Non-Hodgkin lymphoma
(3) Hodgkin lymphoma

Clinical Features
HIV-infected patients often present with enlarged lymph nodes. This may result from viral infections, opportunistic infections or lymphomas of either Hodgkin or non-Hodgkin type. The use of antiretroviral therapy seems, however, to have reduced the incidence of lymphadenopathy in HIV-infected patients. Moreover, the spectrum of lymphoma has also changed as a result of therapy.

Reactive lymphadenopathy in HIV-infected patients is most often localized and massive. In such patients, it is important to use parts of the aspirated material for a wide variety of bacteriological analyses.

HIV patients have a possibly 100-fold risk of developing non-Hodgkin lymphomas, which often present with extranodal manifestations such as CNS, gastrointestinal tract, oral cavity, lung and pleural cavity involvement. Lymphadenopathy is present in less than one third of the patients. The most common subtypes are diffuse large B cell lymphoma, Burkitt/Burkitt-like lymphoma and plasmablastic lymphoma of the oral cavity. However, other subtypes also seem to be overrepresented [1].

The incidence of Hodgkin lymphoma is 5- to 10-fold higher in HIV patients. All subtypes have been described and there is a strong association with EBV [2].

The response to conventional therapy in HIV-infected patients seems to have improved following the introduction of antiretroviral therapy.

Cytology (fig. 7.1)
Lymphadenitis of florid type is a common cause of lymphadenopathy in HIV patients. It is characterized by a heterogeneous population of small, medium-sized and large lymphoid cells as well as plasma cells and tingible body macrophages (fig. 7.1). A large number of immature cells may be suggestive of lymphoma and an immunological characterization is mandatory to verify that the population is reactive. This florid type of hyperplasia will often progress to a depletion phase in which the lymphoid cells are relatively sparse and plasma cells abundant [3–6].

Non-Hodgkin lymphomas are most often of Burkitt or Burkitt-like type but diffuse large B cell type is also relatively common. The cytological diagnosis of the subtypes seldom present any diagnostic difficulties but immunophenotyping should be used to confirm the correct subtyping. The cytomorphology and immunocytochemistry of these entities are described in chapter 4. The plasmablastic variant is characterized by large tumor cells with a basophilic cytoplasm often with a paranuclear clearing. The nucleus is located peripherally and has a distinct nucleolus.

Post-Transplant Lymphoproliferative Disorders

Clinical Features
Patients receiving immunosuppressive therapy after organ transplantation have an increased risk of developing EBV-

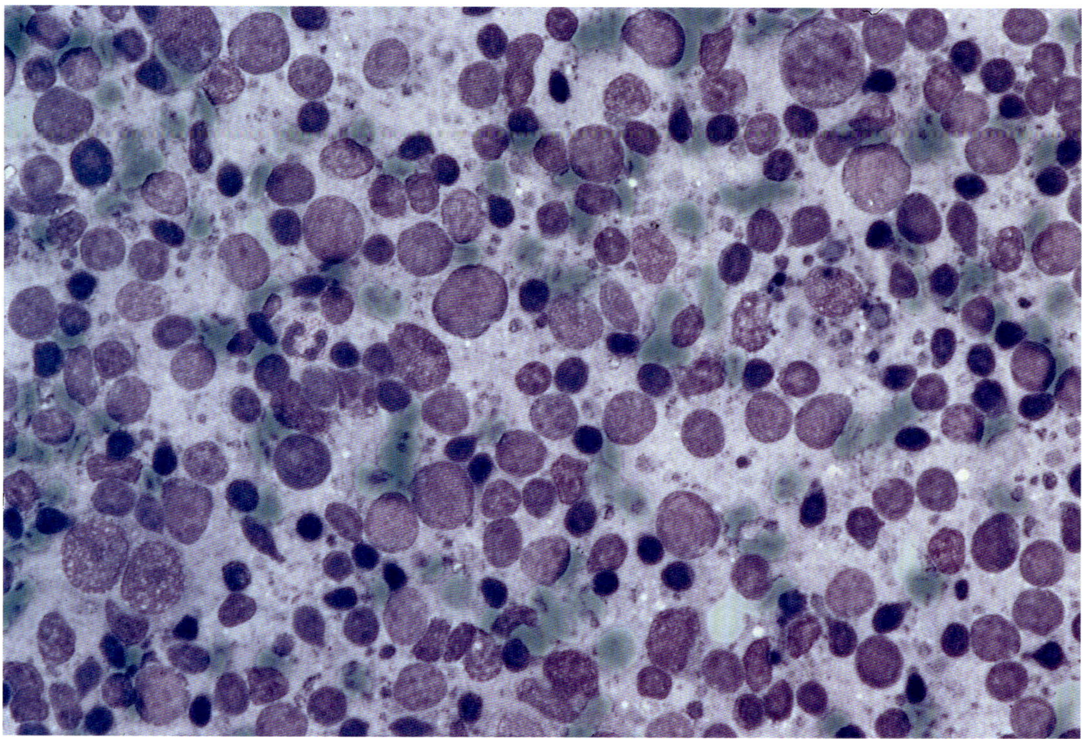

Fig. 7.1. Lymphadenopathy in a HIV-infected patient, hyperplasia of florid type. Smear shows a heterogeneous population of lymphoid cells with the presence of small, medium sized and large immature cells. Few neutrophils and macrophages with apoptotic fragments are found (MGG, high-power view).

Table 7.1. Histologic subtypes of PTLD according to the WHO classification

(1)   Early lesions
      Reactive plasmacytic hyperplasia
      Infectious mononucleosis like
(2)   Polymorphic PTLD
(3)   Monomorphic PTLD
      B cell neoplasms
      Diffuse, large B cell lymphoma (immunoblastic, centroblastic, anaplastic)
      Burkitt/Burkitt-like lymphoma
      Plasma cell myeloma
      Plasmacytoma-like lesions
      T cell neoplasms
      Peripheral T cell lymphoma, not otherwise specified
(4)   Hodgkin lymphoma and Hodgkin lymphoma-like PTLD

associated polyclonal lymphoid proliferation or lymphomas mostly of B phenotype but T cell lymphoma and Hodgkin lymphoma can also occur. The risk varies with type of organ transplant and type of immunosuppressive regimen. For solid organ transplants, the overall risk is around 2% and for marrow recipients it is around 1%. However, the risk is much higher in patients treated for graft vs. host disease. Post-transplant lymphoproliferative disorders (PTLD) often develop in the first years after transplantation but some cases may occur up to 5 years after transplantation [6, 7].

Reduction in immunosuppression usually results in regression of the mononucleosis variant. In monomorphic B or T PTLD, chemotherapy is used in combination with reduction of immunosuppression in most cases. The overall prognosis for monomorphic PTLD is poor [6].

Cytology (fig. 7.2a)

PTLD shows a wide cytologic spectrum reflecting the histologic subtypes according to the WHO classification (table 7.1). Early lesions often mimic mononucleosis while the monomorphic variants of B phenotype can be of the diffuse large cell type, Burkitt-like (fig. 7.2a) or plasmacytoma type. The T cell variants are classified according to the scheme of T cell lymphomas. Hodgkin lymphoma PTLD have been reported to show classical morphologic features [8–13].

Immunocytochemistry (fig. 7.2b): The mononucleosis variant is polyclonal while the monomorphic. B cell variants express the B phenotype (CD19, CD20 and CD79a) and are monoclonal. The EBV-associated antigen LMP-1 is often expressed (fig. 7.2b). The T-PTLDs may express CD4, CD8 or CD30. The Hodgkin variant of PTLD expresses CD15 and CD30.

Immunodeficiency-Associated
Lymphoproliferative Disorders

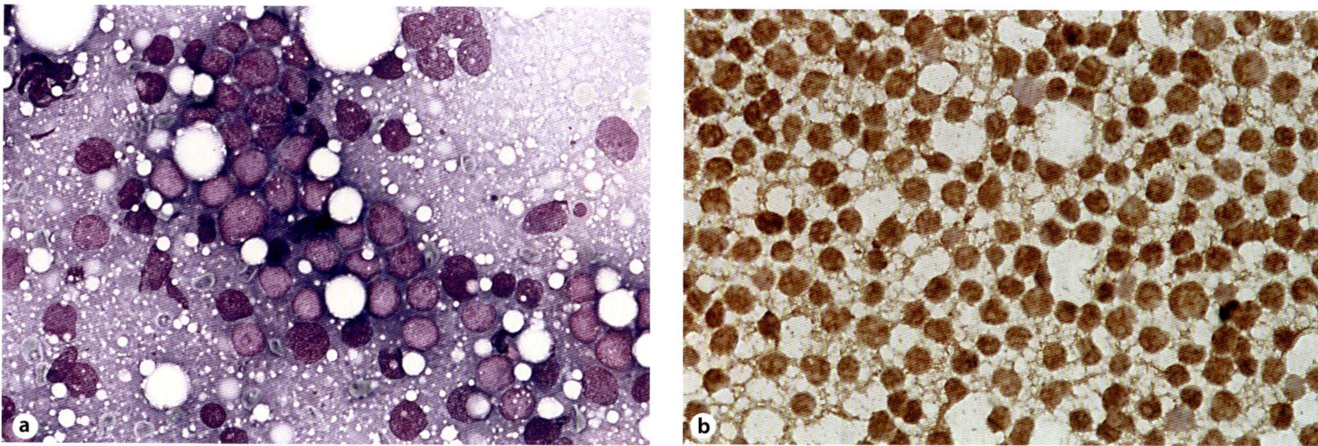

Fig. 7.2. a PTLD. Smear of aspirate from an enlarged lymph node in a patient with renal allograft and immunosuppression. The immature, blastic cells with scant cytoplasm dominate in this Burkitt like variant. MGG, high-power view. **b** PTLD. Aspirate from the same case as in **a** shows EBV-LMP-1 positivity in all tumor cells. immunoperoxidase, high-power view.

References

1 Beral V, Peterman T, Berkelman R, et al: AIDS associated non-Hodgkin lymphoma. Lancet 1991;337:805–809.
2 Goedert JJ: The epidemiology of acquired immunodeficiency syndrome malignancies. Semin Oncol 2000;27:390–401.
3 Reid AJ, Miller RF, Kocjan GI: Diagnostic utility of fine-needle aspiration (FNA) cytology in HIV-infected patients with lymphadenopathy. Cytopathology 1998;9:230–239.
4 Saikia UN, Dey P, Jindal B, et al: Fine needle aspiration cytology in lymphadenopathy of HIV positive cases. Acta Cytol 2001;45:589–592.
5 Nayak S, Mani R, Kavatar AN, et al: Fine needle aspiration cytology in lymphadenopathy of HIV-positive patients. Diagn Cytopathol 2003; 29:146–148.
6 Harris NL, Swerdlow SH, Frizzera G, et al: In Jaffe ES, Harris NL, Stein H, Vardiman JW (eds): World Health Organization Classification of Tumors. Pathology and Genetics of Tumours of Haematopoetic and Lymphoid Tissues. Lyon, IARC Press, 2001.
7 Gattuso P, Manosca F: Fine-needle aspiration of posttransplant lymphoproliferative disorders: a review. Diagn Cytopathol 2005;33: 273–278.
8 Reyes CV, Jensen JA, Chinoy M: Pulmonary lymphoma in cardiac transplant patients treated with OKT3 for rejection: diagnosis by fine-needle aspiration. Diagn Cytopathol 1995;12: 32–36.
9 Dusenbery D, Nalesnik MA, Locker J, Swerdlow SH: Cytologic features of post-transplant lymphoproliferative disorder. Diagn Cytopathol 1997;16:489–496.
10 Gattuso P, Castelli MJ, Peng Y, Reddy VB: Posttransplant lymphoproliferative disorders: a fine-needle aspiration biopsy study. Diagn Cytopathol 1997;16:392–395.
11 Collins BT, Ramos RR, Grosso LE: Combined fine needle aspiration biopsy, and immunophenotypic and genotypic approach to posttransplantation lymphoproliferative disorders. Acta Cytol 1998;42:869–874.
12 Gattuso P, Reddy VB, Kizilbash N, Kluskens L, Selvaggi SM: Role of fine-needle aspiration in the clinical management of solid organ transplant recipients: a review. Cancer 1999; 87:286–294.
13 Hecht JL, Cibas ES, Kutok JL: Fine-needle aspiration cytology of lymphoproliferative disorders in the immunosuppressed patient: the diagnostic utility of in situ hybridization for Epstein-Barr virus. Diagn Cytopathol 2002; 26:360–365.

Immunodeficiency-Associated
Lymphoproliferative Disorders

Chapter 8

Histiocytic and Dendritic Neoplasms

WHO Histological Classification of Histocytic and Dendritic Neoplasms

* Langerhans cell histiocytosis
  Langerhans cell sarcoma
* Histiocytic sarcoma
* Interdigitating/follicular dendritic cell sarcoma[1]/tumor[2]
  Dendritic cell sarcoma, not otherwise specified
(* Indicates subtypes described)

These are very rare neoplasms except for Langerhans cell histiocytosis. In our lymphoma series, we have only one case of histiocytic sarcoma and one of follicular dendritic cell sarcoma which have been verified by histopathology. There are only few case reports on the cytology of interdigitating/ follicular dendritic cell sarcomas.

Langerhans Cell Histiocytosis

Clinical Features
Most of the patients are children but young adults and even middle-aged persons may be affected. Two subgroups exist:

(1) The unifocal type (solitary eosinophilic granuloma), which often involves bone but may occur in lymph node or lung.

(2) The multifocal type which can be unisystemic (Hand-Schüller-Christian disease) or multisystemic (Letterer-Siwe disease). Hand-Schüller-Christian disease involves bone, while Letterer-Siwe may affect bone, skin and liver (fig. 8.1a). The unifocal type has a very good prognosis and spontaneous regression has been described. The multisystemic variant has a poor prognosis [1, 2].

Cytology (fig. 8.1b–d)
The Langerhans cell has an abundant, often pale cytoplasm (MGG) and an oval, grooved nucleus. In addition,

giant cells, eosinophils, neutrophils, histiocytes and lymphocytes are present in varying number. Necrosis may occur. The cytologic presentation in lymph nodes is similar to that of other sites [3–10].

Immunocytochemistry (fig. 8.1e): The cells are CD1a, S-100 and vimentin positive. CD68 and CD45 are often weakly expressed. The rate of cell proliferation is seldom above 20% as measured by MIB-1 staining.

Genetics: A monoclonal proliferation has been demonstrated with analysis of the androgen receptor.

Histiocytic Sarcoma

Clinical Features
All ages can be affected but adults dominate. Lymph nodes, skin and intestinal tract involvement occur. Systemic

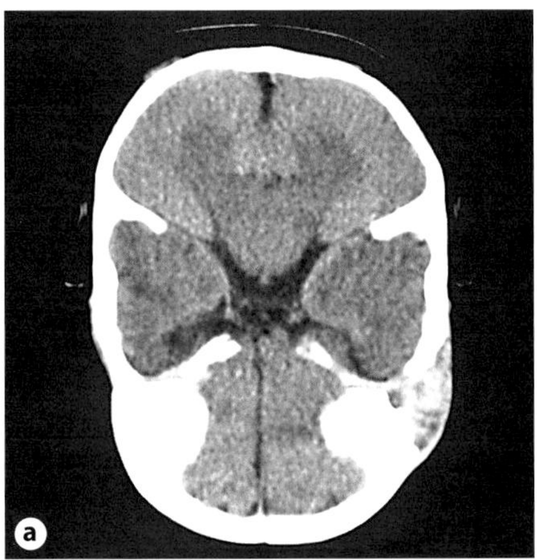

Fig. 8.1. a Langerhans cell histiocytosis. CT shows destruction and engagement of the temporal bone. Courtesy of Dr. Veli Söderlund, Clinical Radiology, Karolinska University Hospital.

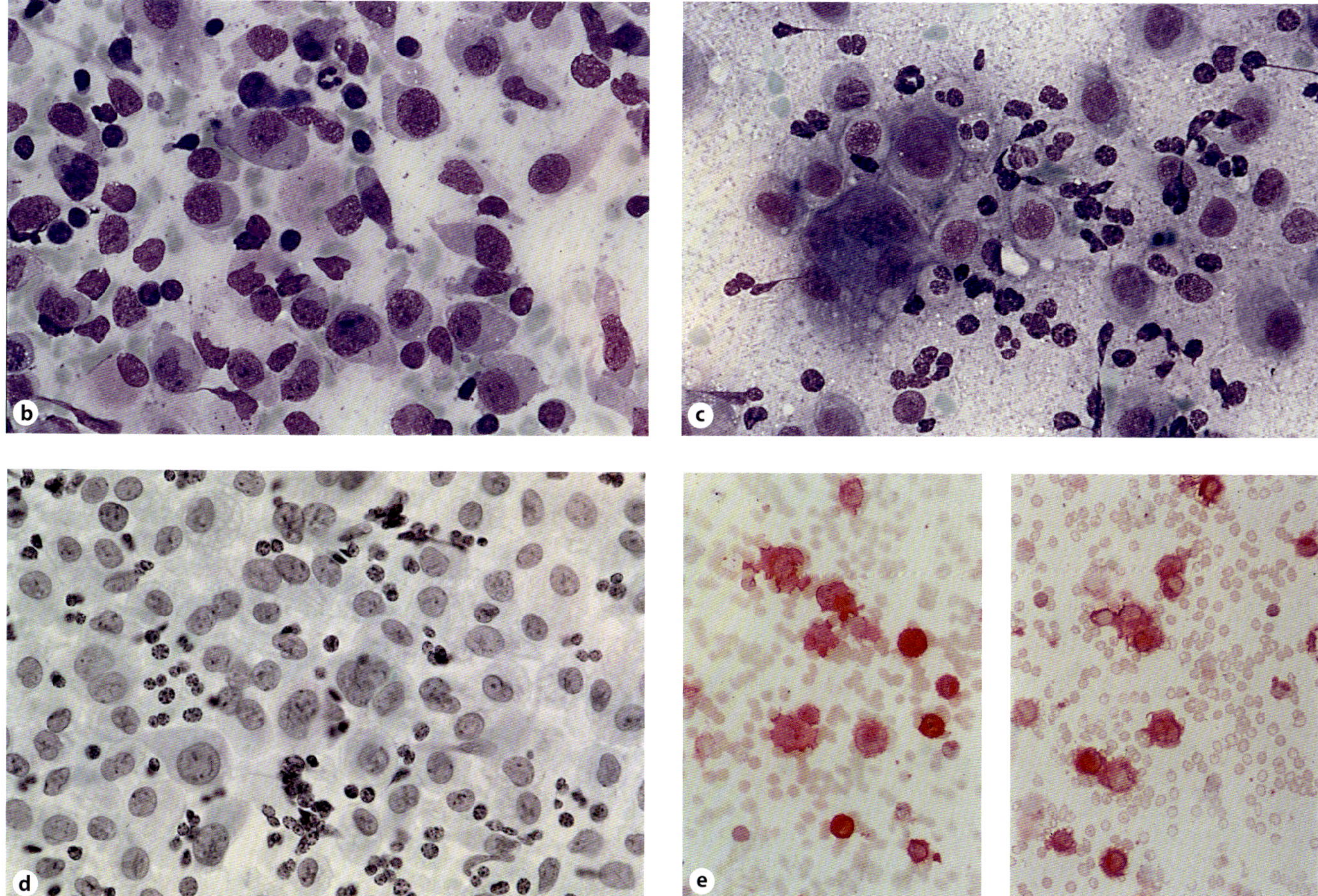

Fig. 8.1 b Langerhans cell histiocytosis. Smear shows polymorphic tumor cells with abundant cytoplasm with oval nuclei, some of 'coffee bean' type. Few lymphocytes and eosinophil granulocytes are present. MGG, high-power view. **c** Langerhans cell histiocytosis. Aspirate shows lymphocytes, eosinophils, histiocytic tumor cells and one multinucleated giant cell. (MGG, high-power view. **d** Langerhans cell histiocytosis. Same aspirate as in **b**. The nuclei are polymorphic and have nuclear grooves. Papanicolaou, high-power view. **e** Langerhans cell histiocytosis. Cytospin preparation from same aspirate as in **d**. CD1a and S100 positivity in the tumor cells. Alkaline phosphatases, medium-power view.

symptoms such as fever and pancytopenia are frequent. The response to therapy is variable but the overall prognosis is poor [11].

Cytology (fig. 8.2a)

The tumor cells are large elongated with round-to-oval nuclei but pleomorphic nuclei can occur. Distinct nucleoli are seen. The cytoplasm is abundant and grey-blue (MGG). Eosinophils, plasma cells, histiocytes and small lymphocytes are present in variable number [4, 12–14].

Immunocytochemistry: Histiocytic markers such as, CD68, lysozyme, CD11c and CD14 are expressed (fig. 8.2b). In addition, CD45 and S-100 are positive. The rate of cell proliferation is highly variable.

Interdigitating/Follicular Dendritic Cell Sarcoma

Clinical Features

These rare tumors occur in adults. Cervical lymph nodes are most often affected but other sites as well as extranodal manifestations occur. The most common presenting symptom is a tumor mass. Systemic symptoms such as fever and fatigue may be present in patients with interdigitating dendritic sarcoma. The prognosis seems to be good for localized disease but patients with widespread tumors seldom survive.

Cytology (fig. 8.3)

The interdigitating tumor cells are large with round vesicular nuclei with distinct nucleoli. There is an abundant

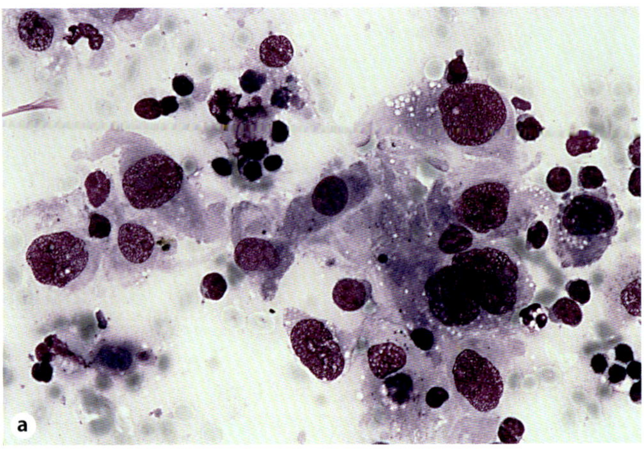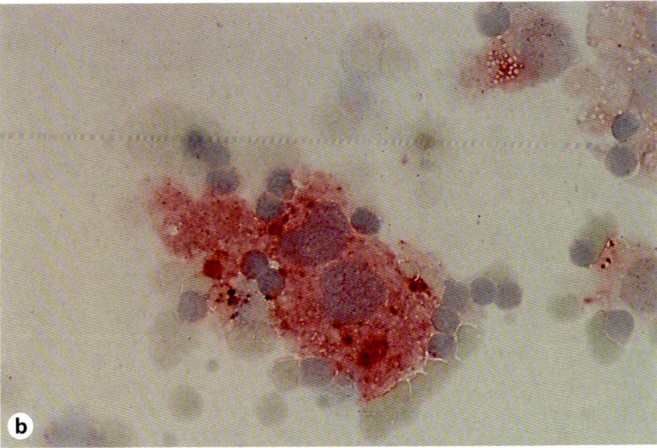

Fig. 8.2. a Histiocytic sarcoma. Smear shows pleomorphic mostly spindle shaped tumor cells with abundant cytoplasm with small vaucoles. MGG, high-power view. **b** Histiocytic sarcoma. Cytospin from same aspirate as in **a** shows tumor cells positive to CD68. Alkaline phosphatase, high-power view.

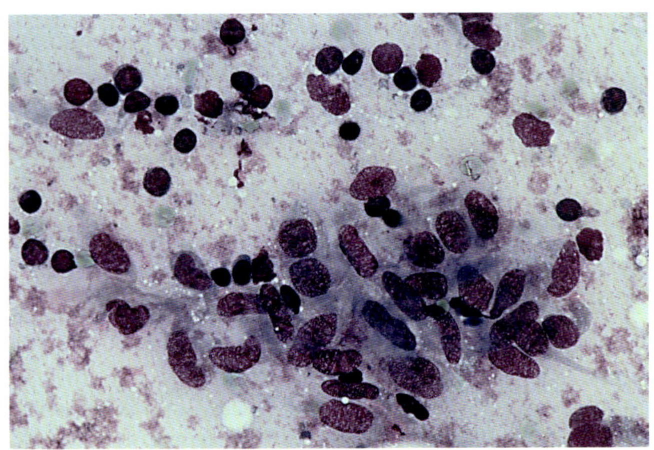

Fig. 8.3. Follicular dendritic tumor. Lymph node aspirate. Tumor cells with elongated/oval nuclei and poorly defined grey/blue cytoplasm mixed with few mature lymphocytes. MGG, high-power view.

admixture of benign lymphoid cells, both of small mature type and of follicular origin, and of eosinophils and plasma cells [15, 16].

Follicular dendritic tumor cells have elongated/oval nuclei with dispersed chromatin and small nucleoli (fig. 8.3). The cytoplasm is abundant and fragile. Small mature lymphocytes are often present [17, 18].

Immunocytochemistry: The interdigitating tumor cells are S100 and vimentin positive. CD45 and CD68 are usually weakly positive. CD1a is not expressed. The follicular dendritic tumor cells are CD21, CD35 or CD23 positive. Vimentin is also positive, while S100 and CD68 are variably positive.

References

1 Lieberman PH, Jones CR, Steinman RM, et al: Langerhans cell (eosinophilic) granulomatosis: a clinico-pathologic study encompassing 50 years. Am J Surg Pathol 1996;20:519–552.

2 Greenberger JS, Crocke AC, Crocke AC, Vawter G, et al: Results of treatment of 127 patients with systemic histiocytosis (Letterer-Siwe syndrome, Schüller-Christian syndrome and multifocal eosinophilic granuloma). Medicine (Baltimore) 1981;60:311–338.

3 Das D: Lymph nodes; in Bibbo M (ed): Comprehensive Cytopathology, ed 2. Philadelphia, Saunders, 1997, pp 703–731.

4 Orell S, Sterrett G, Whitaker D, van Heerde P, Miliauskas J: Lymph nodes; in Orell S, Sterrett G, Whitaker D (eds): Fine Needle Aspiration Cytology, ed 5. London, Churchill-Livingstone, 2005, pp 83–124.

    Histiocytic and Dendritic Neoplasms

5 Kocjan G: Lymph nodes; in Kocjan G (ed): Clinical Cytopathology of the Head and Neck. London, Greenwich Medical Media, 2001.
6 Van Heerde P, Maarten Egler R: The cytology of Langerhans cell histiocytosis (histiocytosis X). Cytopathology 1991;2:149–158.
7 Pohar-Marmsek Z, Us-Krasovec M: Cytomorphology of Langerhans cell histiocytosis. Acta Cytol 1996;40:1257–1264.
8 Lee JS, Lee MC, Park CS, et al: Fine needle aspiration cytology of Langerhans-cell histiocytosis confined to lymph node: a case report. Acta Cytol 1997;41:1793–1796.
9 Kakkar S, Kapila K, Verma K: Langerhans cell histiocytosis in lymph nodes: cytomorphologic diagnosis and pitfalls. Acta Cytol 2001;45: 327–332.
10 Bhadani PP, Sah SP, Agarwal A, Tewari A: Fine needle aspiration diagnosis of congenital Langerhans cell histiocytosis of the lymph nodes with isolated skin involvement. Acta Cytol 2005;49:114–116.
11 Soria C, Orradre JL, Garcia-Almagro D, et al: True histiocytic lymphoma (monocytic sarcoma). Am J Dermatopathol 1992;14:511–517.
12 Bizjak-Schwarzbartl M: Color Atlas of Non-Hodgkin's Lymphoma: Fine Needle Aspiration Biopsy. Ljubljana, Institute of Oncology, 1994.
13 van Heerde P, Meyer CJLM, Noorduyn LA, van der Valk P: An Atlas and Textbook of Malignant Lymphomas: Cytology, Histopathology and Immunocytochemistry. London, Harvey Miller, Oxford University Press, 1996.
14 Miliauskas JR: Fine-needle aspiration cytology: true histiocytic lymphoma/histiocytic sarcoma. Diagn Cytopathol 2003;29:233–235.
15 Ylagan LR, Bartlett NL, Kraus M: Interdigitating dendritic reticulum cell tumor of lymph nodes: case report with differential diagnostic considerations. Diagn Cytopathol 2003;28:278–281.
16 Jayaram G, Mun KS, Elsayed EM, et al: Interdigitating dendritic reticulum cell sarcoma: cytologic, histologic and immunocytochemical features. Diagn Cytopathol 2005; 33:43–48.
17 Wright CA, Nayler SJ, Leiman G: Cytopathology of follicular dendritic cell tumors. Diagn Cytopathol 1997;17:138–142.
18 Mohanty SK, Dey P, Vashishta RK, Rajwanshi A: Cytologic diagnosis of follicular dendritic cell tumor: a diagnostic dilemma. Diagn Cytopathol 2003;29:368–369.

Chapter 9

Extranodal Lymphomas

Some lymphoma subtypes such as extranodal marginal zone B cell lymphoma, primary cutaneous B cell lymphoma, plasmablastic lymphoma of the oral cavity, primary cutaneous anaplastic large cell lymphoma extranodal NK/T cell lymphoma nasal type and primary effusion lymphoma are almost exclusively extranodal in their initial phase [1, 2].

Other subtypes such as:

(1) marginal zone B cell lymphoma of mucosa associated tissue (MALT lymphoma),
(2) Burkitt lymphoma,
(3) cutaneous T cell lymphoma (mycosis fungoides, Sézary syndrome, primary cutaneous anaplastic large cell lymphoma),
(4) extranodal NK/T cell lymphoma nasal type, and
(5) primary cutaneous anaplastic large cell lymphoma

show a predilection for extranodal growth but nodal engagement is not rare. They have already been described in chapters 4 and 5.

In contrast, other subtypes can, rarely, be present exclusively in extranodal sites such as the gastrointestinal tract, thyroid, skin, orbit, salivary glands, bone, lung, kidney,

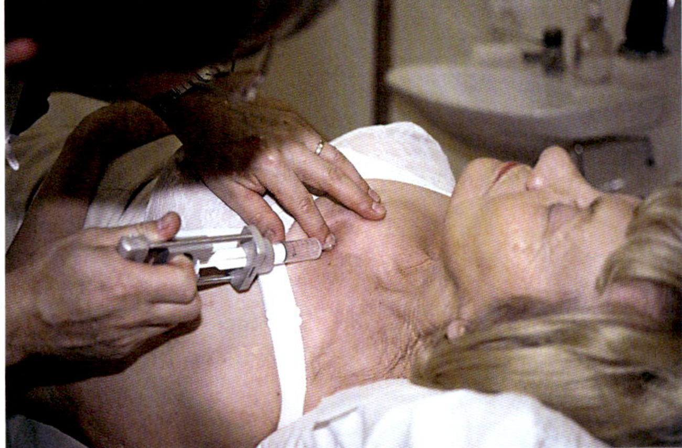

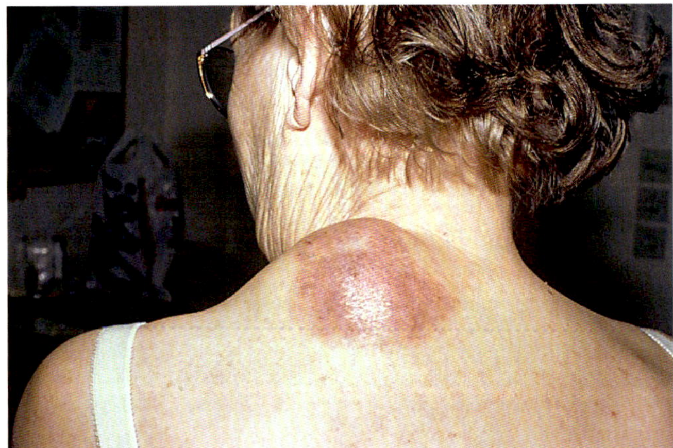

Fig. 9.1. Primary nodal lymphomas with tumorous extranodal manifestations.

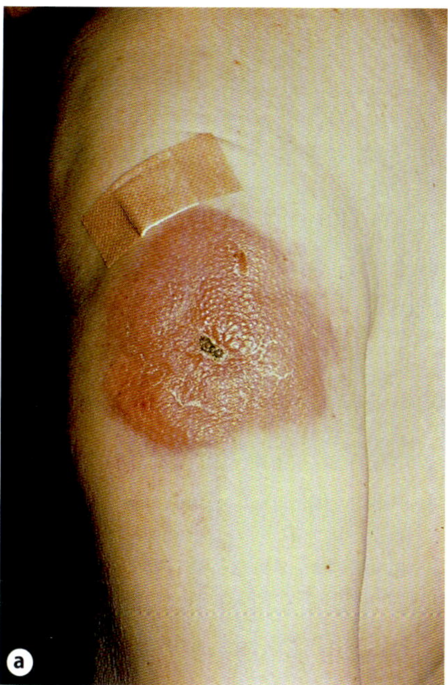

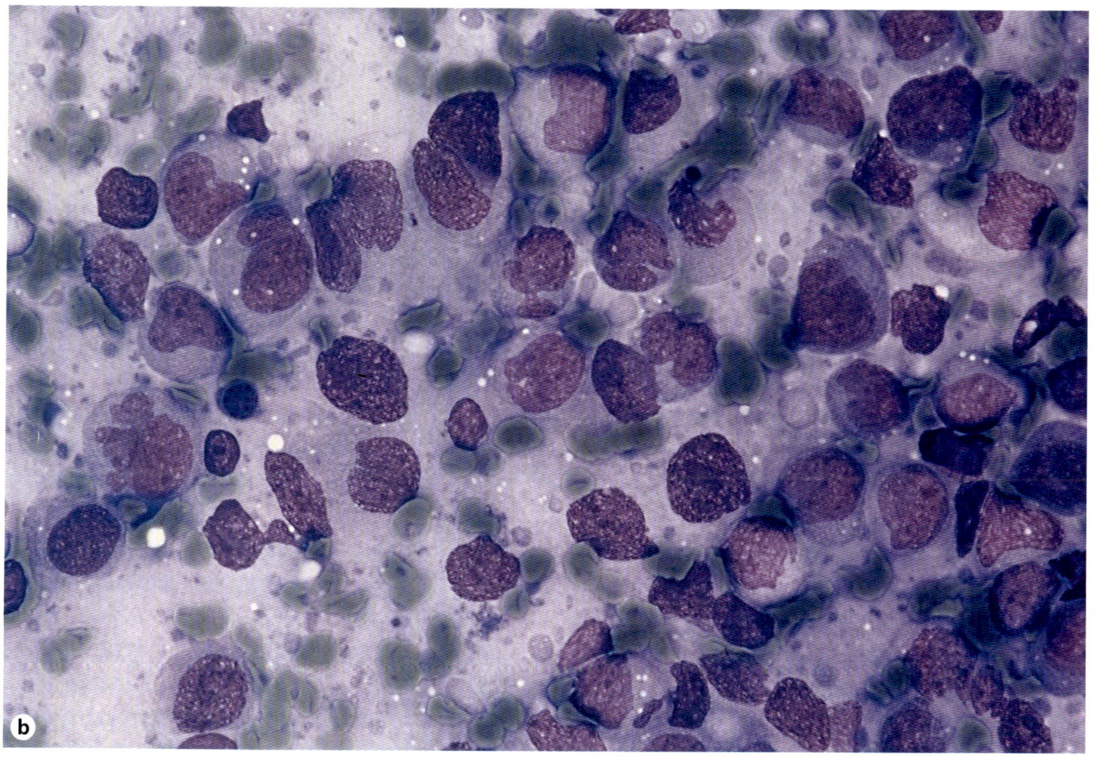

Fig. 9.2. a Primary cutaneous lymphoma. A large erythematous infiltrate. **b** Primary cutaneous lymphoma. Smear from the lesion shown in **a** presents with immature lymphatic cells with irregular polymorphic cells. MGG, high-power view.

gonads and CNS [1–8]. However, many primarily nodal lymphomas eventually progress to secondarily involve extranodal sites (fig. 9.1). The cytologic presentation of various lymphomas at the extranodal sites is similar to that of FNA smears from the lymph nodes.

The following entities are described in this chapter:
(1) Primary cutaneous B cell lymphoma
(2) Primary effusion lymphoma
(3) Plasmablastic lymphoma of the oral cavity

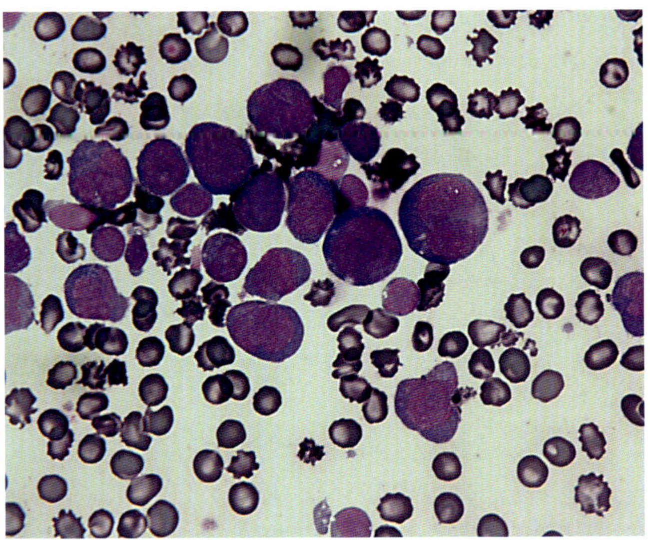

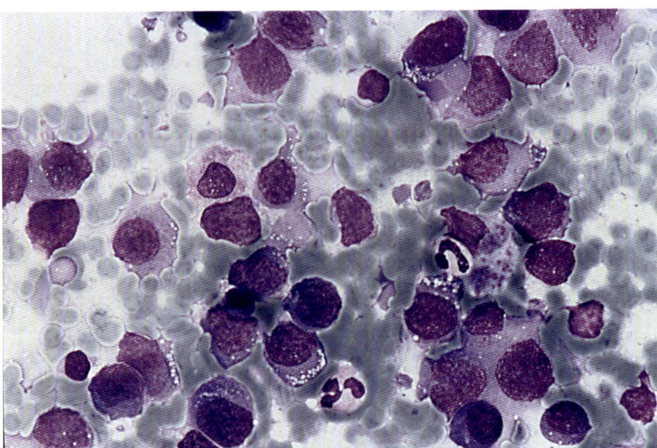

Fig. 9.4. Plasmablastic lymphoma of the oral cavity. Aspiration smear shows large immature cells with eccentric nuclei with coarse chromatin and small vacuoles in the cytoplasm. Few cells with plasma cell differentiation are seen. MGG, high-power view.

Fig. 9.3. Primary effusion lymphoma. MGG, high-power view. Courtesy of Jean-Louis Dargent, l'Institut J. Bordet, Brussels, Belgium.

Primary Cutaneous B Cell Lymphoma

Clinical Features (fig. 9.2a)

The follicular variant generally occurs on the trunk or head. The large cell type involves the skin of the extremities [2]. The follicular variant responds to local therapy and has an excellent prognosis. The diffuse subtype has a distinctly worse prognosis.

Cytology (fig. 9.2b)

The follicular variant is composed of centrocytes and centroblasts in varying proportions and the cytology is identical to that of nodal follicle center lymphoma. It is not possible to identify the follicular pattern on smears and the cytologic diagnosis will be follicle centre lymphoma. The large cell variant is dominated by centroblasts and sometimes by immunoblasts (fig. 9.2b).

Immunology

The follicular variants show light chain restriction and are CD20 and Bcl-6+, CD10−/+ and bcl-2−. The large cell variant express CD20, bcl-2, bcl-6+ but not CD10.

Cytogenetics: t[14;18] is not found.

Primary Effusion Lymphoma

Clinical Features

This is a rare entity occurring in HIV-positive patients [2, 8]. It typically presents in pleural or peritoneal effusions but concomitant solid tumors may occur. The prognosis is poor [8].

Cytology (fig. 9.3)

The tumor cell can be of immunoblastic type but anaplastic variants have been described.

Immunology

The cells are CD45+, CD138+, CD30+ and CD38+. CD20 and CD79 are not expressed.

Plasmablastic Lymphoma of the Oral Cavity

Clinical Features

This entity is found almost exclusively in HIV-infected patients [8]. The oral mucosa and/or jaw are the sites afflicted with this rapidly growing tumor. The response to therapy is good.

Cytology (fig. 9.4)

The tumor cells are large with an eccentrically placed nucleus with a large nucleolus.

Immunocytochemistry: CD138 and LMP-1 positivity is observed. There is no expression of CD20 and CD79a.

References

1 Burke JS: The diagnosis of extranodal lymphomas and lymphoid hyperplasias ('pseudolymphomas') other than those involvning the lung; in Jaffe ES (ed): Surgical Pathology of the Lymph Nodes and Related Organs. Philadelphia, Saunders, 1985, pp 298–328.
2 Campo E, Chott A, Kinney MC, et al: Update on extranodal lymphomas. Conclusions of the workshop held by the EAHP and the SH in Thessaloniki, Greece. Histopathology 2006;48: 481–504.
3 Longerich T, Schirmacher P, Dienes HP, et al: Malignant lymphomas of the liver: new diagnostic algorithms. Pathologe 2006;27:263–272.
4 Battula N, Srinivasan P, Prachialias A, et al: Primary pancreatic lymphoma: diagnostic and therapeutic dilemma. Pancreas 2006;33: 192–194.
5 Sanchez M, Hebrero ML, Mesa C, et al: Primary bone lymphoma. Clin Transl Oncol 2006;8:221–224.
6 Descamps MJ, Barrett L, Groves M, et al: Primary sciatic nerve lymphoma: a case report and review of the literature. J Neurol Neurosurg Psychiatry 2006;77:1087–1089.
7 Batchelor T, Loeffler JS: Primary CNS lymphoma. J Clin Oncol 2006;24:1281–1288.
8 Raphael M, Borisch B, Jaffe ES: Lymphoma associated with infection by the human immune deficiency virus (HIV); in Jaffe ES, Harris NL, Stein H, Vardiman JW (eds): World Health Organization Classification of Tumors. Pathology and Genetics of Tumors of Haematopoetic and Lymphoid Tissues. Lyon, IARC Press, 2001, pp 260–263.

Chapter 10

Lymphoma Look-Alike

Lesions that Cytologically Can Be Mistaken for Lymphoma

* Reactive lymphadenopathy
* Sinus histiocytosis with massive lymphadenopathy
* Acute myeloid lymphoblastic leukemia
* Cutaneous B cell pseudolymphoma
* Poorly differentiated carcinoma
* Merkel cell carcinoma
* Malignant melanoma
* Seminoma/dysgerminoma
* Desmoplastic round cell tumor
* Ewing's sarcoma
* Neuroblastoma
* Rhabdomyosarcoma
* Wilms' tumor
(* Indicates entities described)

Reactive Lymphadenopathy

Clinical Features (fig. 10.1a)

Marked enlargement of lymph nodes can be seen in a variety of conditions such as (1) reactive follicular hyperplasia as a response to local infection, rheumatoid arthritis, systemic lupus erythematosus and HIV infection, and (2) paracortical hyperplasia which most often follows viral infections such as infectious mononucleosis but may be induced by medication or vaccination. In many cases of reactive hyperplasia, the two types, follicular and paracortical hyperplasia, are present together.

Cytology (fig. 10.1b, c)

In aspirates from most cases of follicular hyperplasia, the entire spectrum of lymphoid cells is present albeit in variable numbers. Small mature lymphocytes, centrocytes and centroblasts can easily be identified. Macrophages with tingible bodies are always present. Plasma cells can often be found. In extreme cases, the medium-sized or large cells dominate to such an extent that a high-grade lymphoma cannot be excluded. An immunologic characterization of the lymphoid population should be carried out to corroborate the cytologic diagnosis [1–7].

Aspirates from paracortical hyperplasia show small mature lymphoid cells, plasma cells and numerous immunoblasts which may dominate the smears (fig. 10.1c). In rare cases, the immunoblasts may show irregular nuclei and prominent nucleoli which thus can mimic T cell lymphoma or even Hodgkin lymphoma [1–9].

Immunocytochemistry: CD4 and CD8 T cells are present with a ratio varying from 1.6 to 7.4. The B cells are polyclonal with few cells express CD10 and BCL-2. In paracortical hyperplasia, the immunoblast may express CD30 but they always express CD45 and T or B cell markers, which excludes Hodgkin lymphoma.

Genetics: In extreme cases of follicular hyperplasia, Ig gene rearrangement has to be excluded. In paracortical hyperplasia there is no rearrangement of the T cell receptor.

Sinus Histiocytosis with Massive Lymphadenopathy (Rosai-Dorfman)

Clinical Features

This disorder is most common in children or young adults of Asian or African origin. Massive cervical lymphadenopathy is usually present as well as fever. The disorder runs a prolonged course but spontaneous regression follows in most cases.

Cytology (fig. 10.2a, b)

Lymphocytes of varying type dominate but large pale histiocytes are easily found. These cells have an abundant

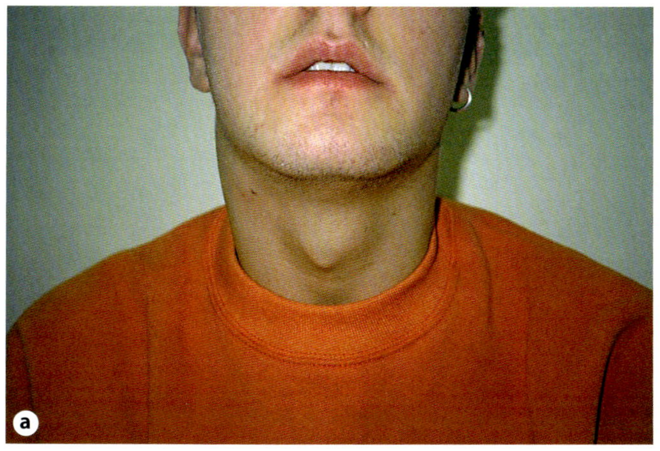

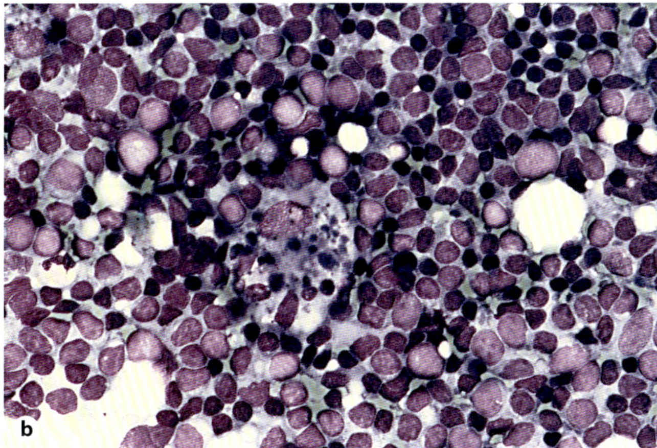

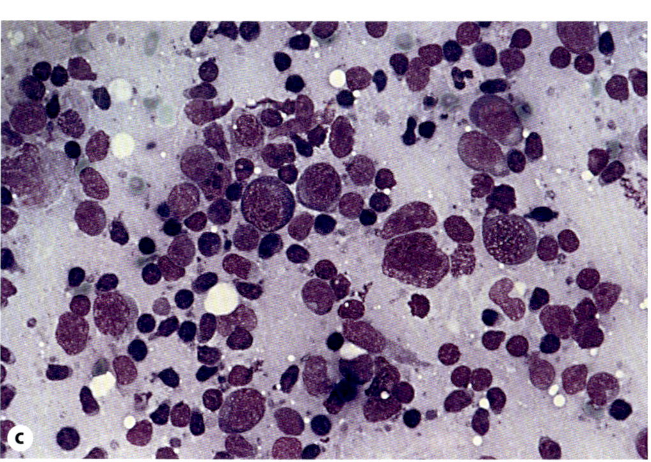

Fig. 10.1. a Reactive lymphadenopathy. Enlarged node in the neck. **b** Reactive lymphadenopathy with follicular hyperplasia. Smear shows mixed small mature lymphocytes and blastic lymphoid cells, few granulocytes and a macrophage with tingible bodies. MGG, high-power view. **c** Reactive lymphadenopathy with paracortical hyperplasia. Smear shows small mature lymphocytes and numerous immunoblasts in a case of infectious mononucleosis. MGG, high-power view.

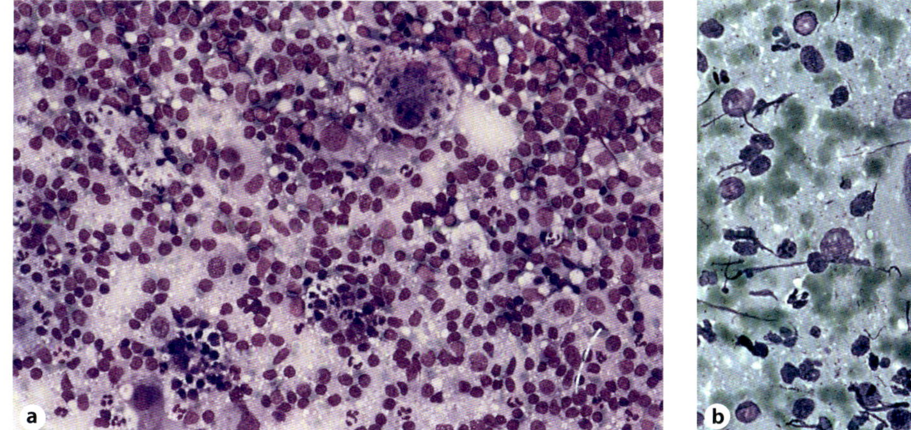

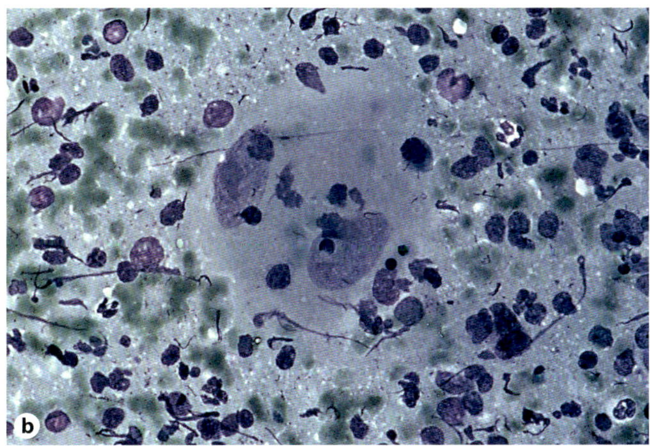

Fig. 10.2. a Sinus histiocytosis with massive lymphadenopathy (Rosai-Dorfman disease). Smear shows predominance of lymphocytes, few granulocytes and presence of large histiocytes with lymphocytes in the cytoplasm (emperipolesis). MGG, medium-power view. **b** Sinus histiocytosis with massive lymphadenopathy (Rosai-Dorfman disease). A binucleated large histiocyte with lymphocytes in the cytoplasm (emperipolesis). MGG, high-power view.

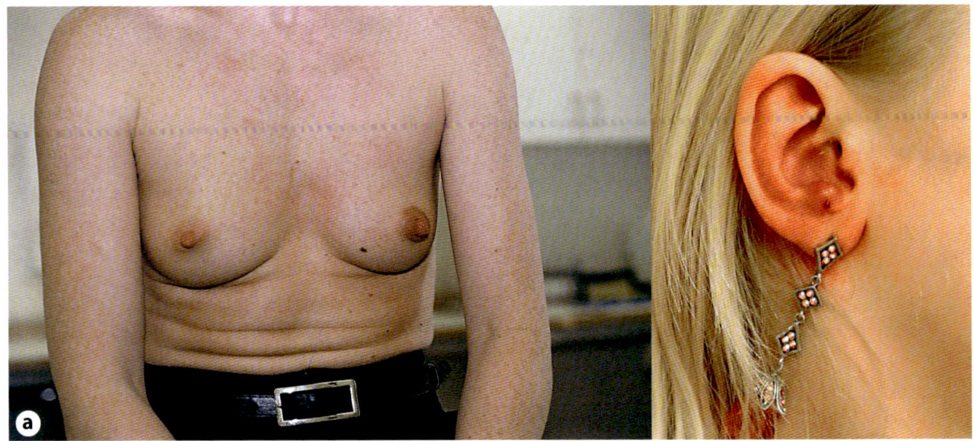

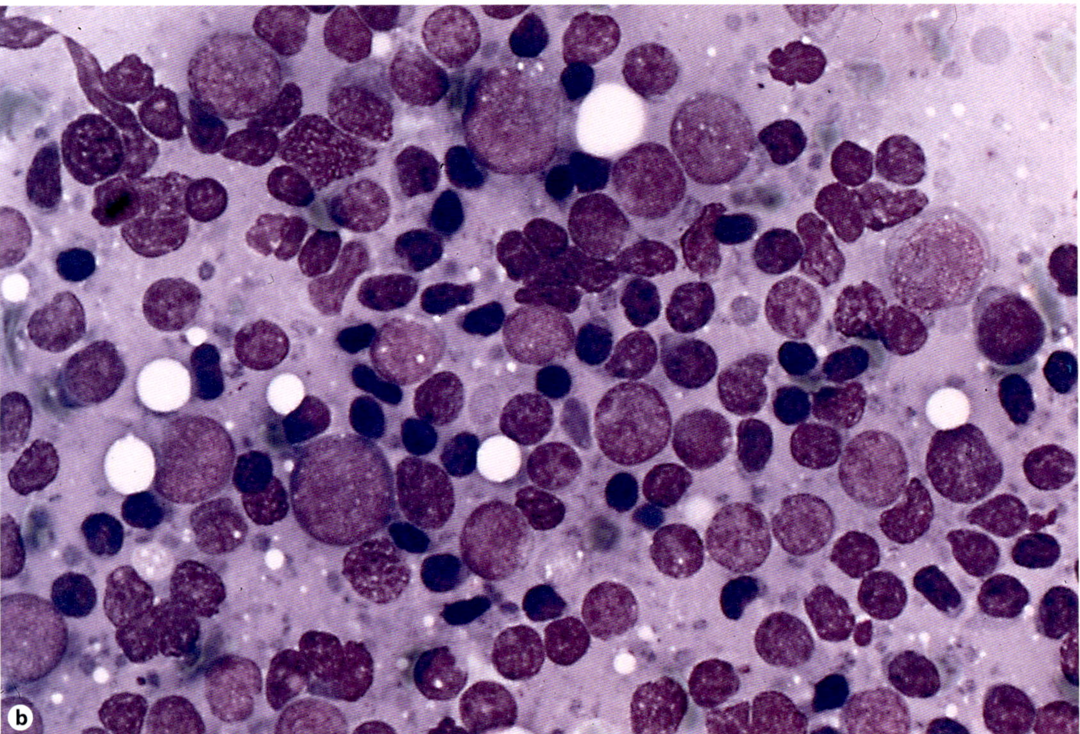

Fig. 10.3. **a** Cutaneous B cell pseudolymphoma. Typical clinical presentation in the ear-lobe (right) and areolae (left). **b** Cutaneous B cell pseudolymphoma. A mixed lymphoid cell population with relatively large number of centroblasts and some immunoblasts. MGG, high-power view.

cytoplasm in which preserved lymphocytes (emperipolesis) are typically present [2–5, 10–14].

Immunocytochemistry: The cytologic presentation is typical and an immunologic characterization is seldom required. The lymphocytes are of T and B phenotype. The histiocytes typically express S-100 and CD68. In addition, lysozyme and MAC 387 are often positive.

Cutaneous B Cell Pseudolymphoma (Lymphadenosis Benigna Cutis)

Clinical Features (fig. 10.3a)

Most patients are adult and females dominate. In a majority of cases, only one site is affected and the lesion is usually elevated and dark blue-brown-red. The most common site of

　Lymphoma Look-Alike

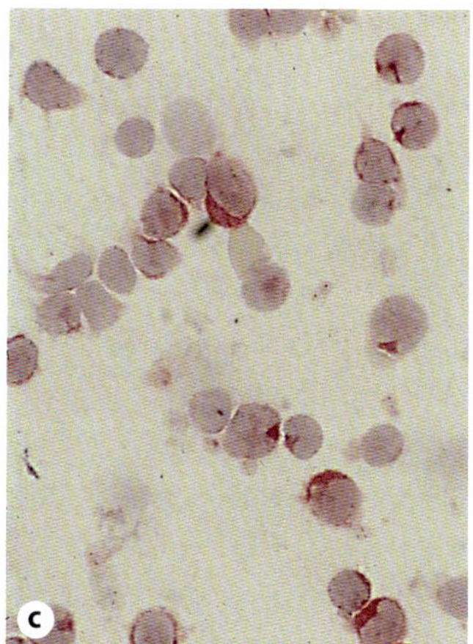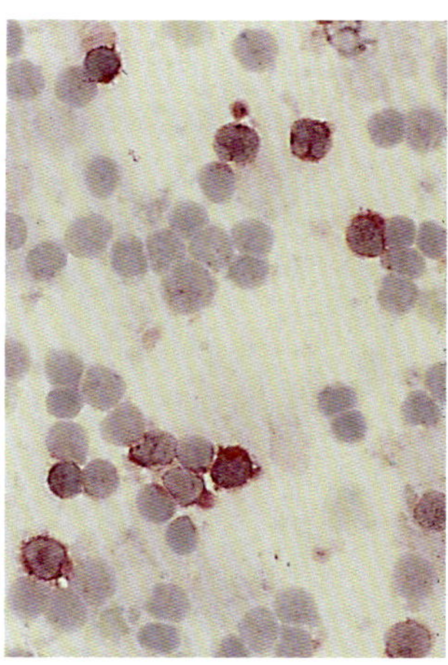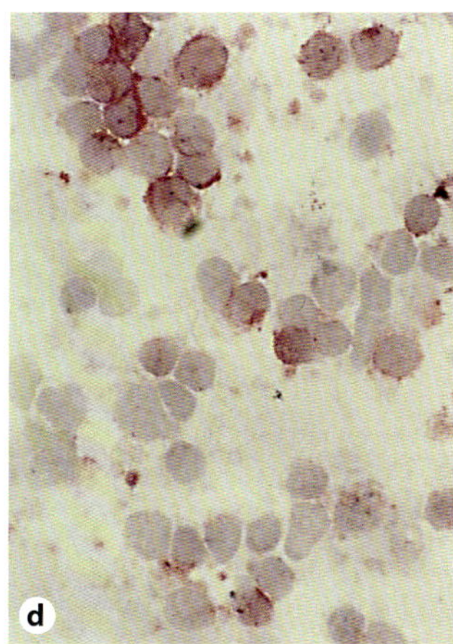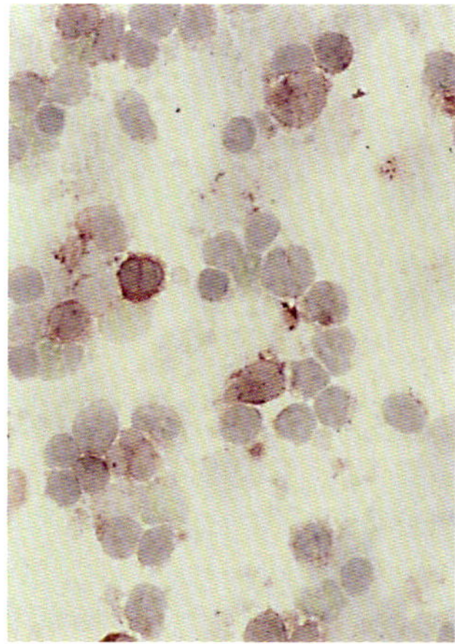

Fig. 10.3. **c** Immunocytochemistry on the same aspirate as **b**. The population is composed of many medium and large-sized B cells (left) and some small T lymphocytes (right). (Alkaline phosphatase, high-power view. **d** Immunocytochemistry on the same aspirate as in **b** and **c** A polyclonal population with kappa (left) and lambda (right) positive B cells (alkaline phosphatase, high-power view).

presentation is the ear lobe, breast areola and scrotum. The patients often have a history of previous tick bite and there is growing evidence that the lesion is caused by a *Borrelia* infection. Penicillin treatment results in cure [15].

Cytology (fig. 10.3b)

The smears can be dominated by centroblasts but small and medium-sized lymphoid cells are always present. Granulocytes and macrophages are scarce. The cytology mimics that of a follicle center cell lymphoma of intermediate or high grade and a conclusive diagnosis requires an immunologic characterization of the cells.

Immunocytochemistry (fig. 10.3c, d): B cells are polyclonal and T cells are mostly mature.

Acute Myeloid/Lymphoblastic Leukemia

Clinical Features (fig. 10.4a)

Nodal and extranodal (soft tissue, bone) manifestation of acute myeloid leukemia (AML) may occur without bone marrow involvement both in patients with or without any previous history of AML. All ages are represented. Most patients with extramedullary AML will develop leukemia sometimes after several years. The prognosis is similar to that of AML although patients with an isolated lesion may experience long survival and even cure has been reported.

In patients with nodal involvement of lymphoblasts, the classification into lymphoma or leukemia depends on the dominant site of involvement. Patients with involved lymph nodes and less than 25% blasts in the marrow are classified as lymphoblastic lymphoma.

Cytology (fig. 10.4b)

The tumor cells are blastic or immature and lineage cannot be determined cytologically. Ancillary techniques are thus required for a conclusive diagnosis [16–18].

Immunocytochemistry (fig. 10.4c): Myeoloblasts express CD13, CD33, CD43 and CD117. Monoblasts are CD11C+, CD14+, CD68+ and CD116+. B cell lymphoblasts are CD19+ and CD79a+, while T cell lymphoblasts are often CD3+ and CD7+.

Metastases

Neoplastic enlargement of lymph nodes caused by metastatic malignancy far outweighs malignant lymphoma. In fact, a lymph node metastasis is often the first clinical manifestation of a malignant neoplasm. Most tumors can spread to lymph nodes but the incidence of lymph node metastasis varies depending on tumor type. Thus, carcinomas and melanomas often spread to regional lymph nodes while mesotheliomas and most sarcomas only rarely spread this way. Secondary deposits in lymph nodes often reproduce features of the primary lesion and are thus readily recognizable. In fact, the primary site can sometimes be inferred from the cytologic features of the metastasis. Examples of this are renal cell carcinoma, and carcinoma of the large bowel, breast and thyroid [19]. More commonly, the lack of specific cytologic features will present a diagnostic problem both

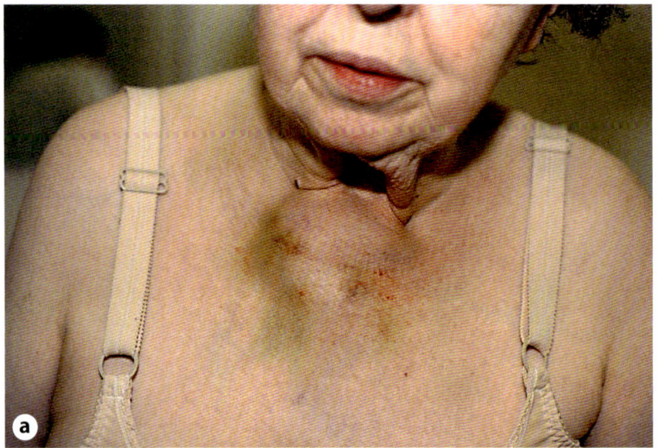

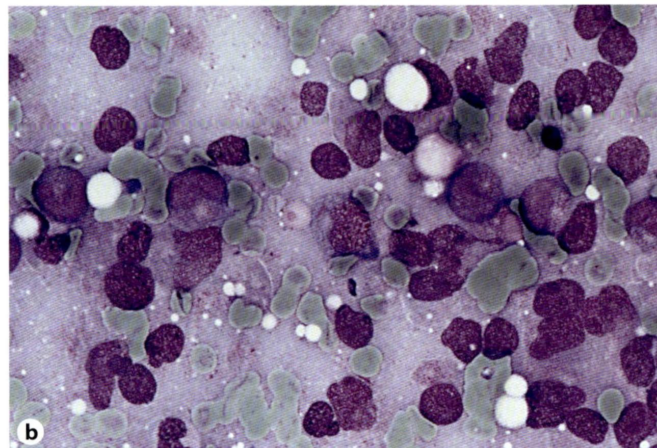

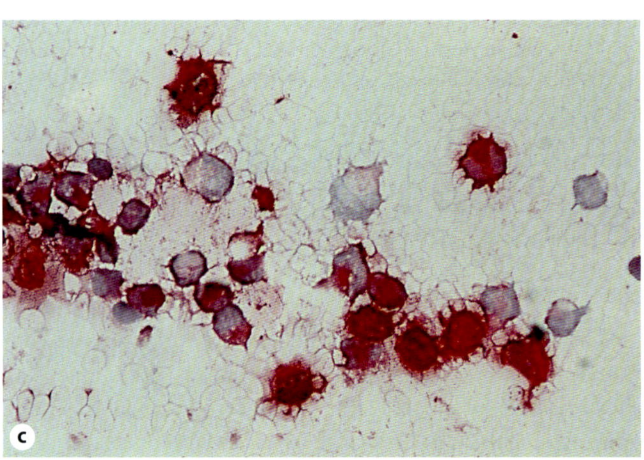

Fig. 10.4. a AML/granulocytic sarcoma. Extranodal manifestation presenting as a presternal tumor. **b** AML/granulocytic sarcoma. Smear from the aspirate of the tumor shown in **a**, immature cells of myeoloic type with fine pink granula in the cytoplasm. MGG, high-power view. **c** AML/granulocytic sarcoma. Immunocytochemistry on the same aspirate as in **b** showing positivity for CD33 (my9). Alkaline phophatase, high-power view.

with respect to classification and identification of primary site. Immunocytochemistry will in many instances aid a more precise cytologic diagnosis and today this technique is indispensable in routine cytology work. In addition, immuno-cytochemistry can demonstrate features of importance for prognosis and choice of treatment.

Poorly Differentiated Carcinoma

The most common 'lymphoma look-alike' epithelial tumor is small cell undifferentiated carcinoma of the lung. However, metastasis from other poorly differentiated carcinomas, e.g. of prostate, lung, ovary, tonsil and epipharynx, may also cause considerable diagnostic difficulties.

Cytologic Features (fig. 10.5a)
The individual cell may show features almost identical to a high-grade lymphoma. However, In cellular smears, there

are, always areas where the abnormal cells show a tendency to cohesion and moulding. The identification of occasional 'lymphoglandular bodies' is not sufficient to diagnose a lymphoma but paranuclear inclusions strongly suggest epithelial origin [19–22]. The cytologic diagnosis should preferably be corroborated by immunocytochemistry.

Immunocytochemistry (fig. 10.5b): Carcinoma cells express CK and/ EMA. CD45 is never expressed. A CD30 positivity can be found in some metastatic tumors such as embryonal carcinoma, salivary duct carcinoma and pancreatic cancer.

Merkel Cell Carcinoma

Clinical Features (fig. 10.6a)
The tumor is often cutaneous/subcutaneous and almost only found in elderly patients. It is highly aggressive and has a strong tendency both to recur locally and to metastasize to regional lymph nodes. Overall survival is poor.

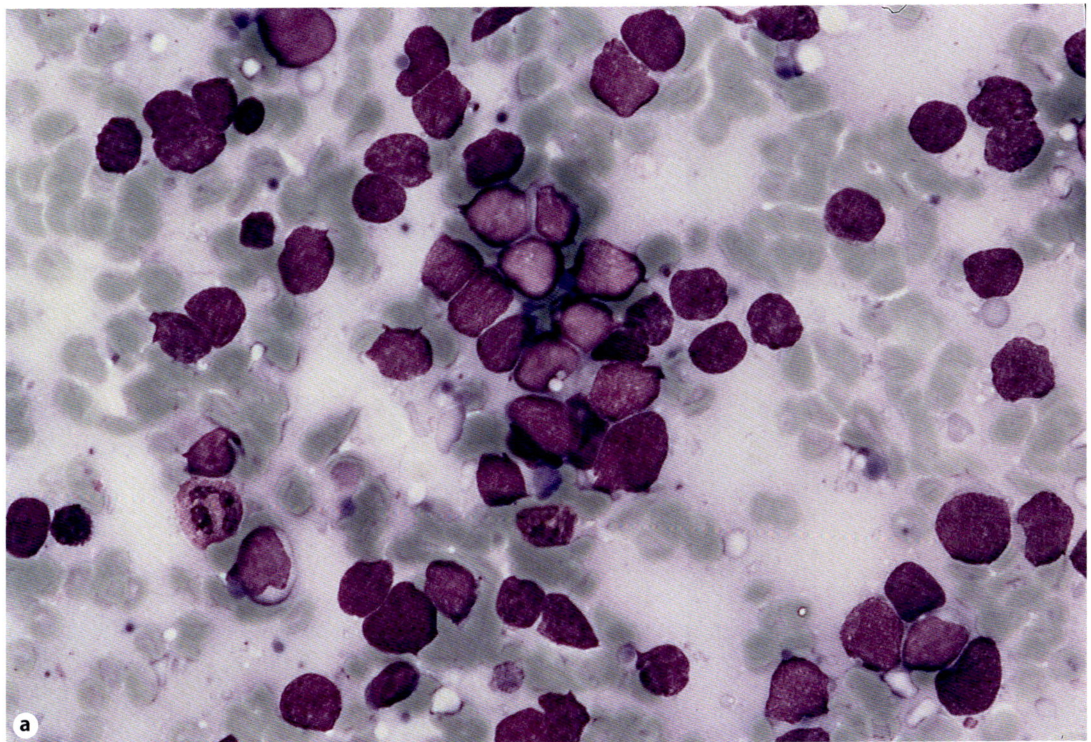

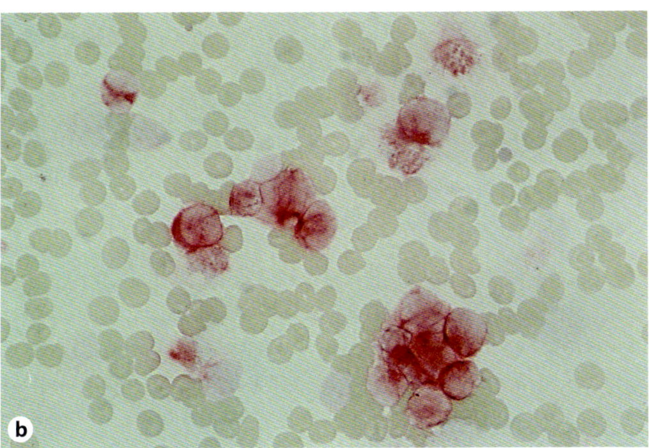

Fig. 10.5. a Poorly differentiated carcinoma. FNA from a lymph-node. Small round tumor cells with scant cytoplasm and a tendency to molding. The cytomorphology lymphoma. MGG, high-power view. **b** Immunocytochemistry performed on the same aspirate as in **a** showing positivity of tumor cells for CK (alkaline phosphatase, high-power view).

Cytologic Features (fig. 10.6b)

The tumor cells are fragile and disrupt easily when smeared but few cytoplasmic fragments can be identified. The cells have a round-to-oval nucleus with bland chromatin and indistinct nucleoli. A small distinct blue inclusion is seen in the nucleus. The sparse cytoplasm is light blue. Cellular moulding is frequent. Mitoses are readily found [23–27].

Immunocytochemistry (fig. 10.6c): The cells are CK+ and CK20+ (dot like) (fig. 10.6c). Most cases express chromogranin and NSE. CK7 and CD45 are always negative.

Malignant Melanoma

The cytologic presentation of metastatic melanoma may vary considerably both between patients and in different lesions in the same patient. The diagnosis of metastatic melanoma is often easy because of a typical cytomorphologic presentation and a past history of melanoma.

However, cytologically, metastatic melanoma sometimes mimics other tumors to such an extent that a conclusive diagnosis requires an immunologic characterization of the cells.

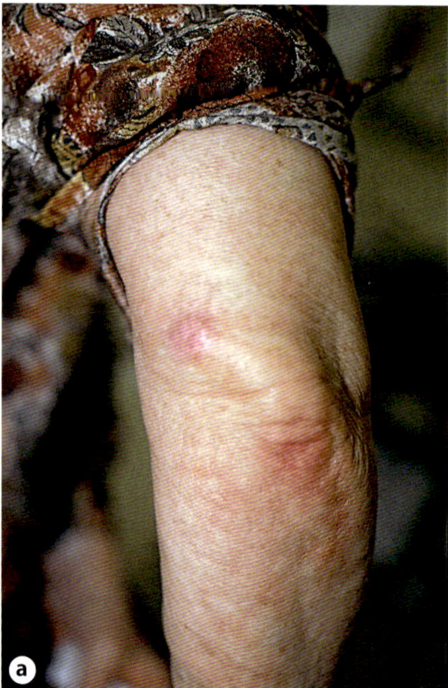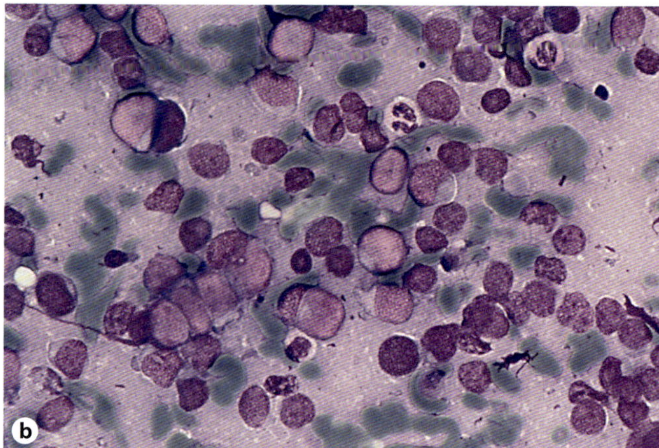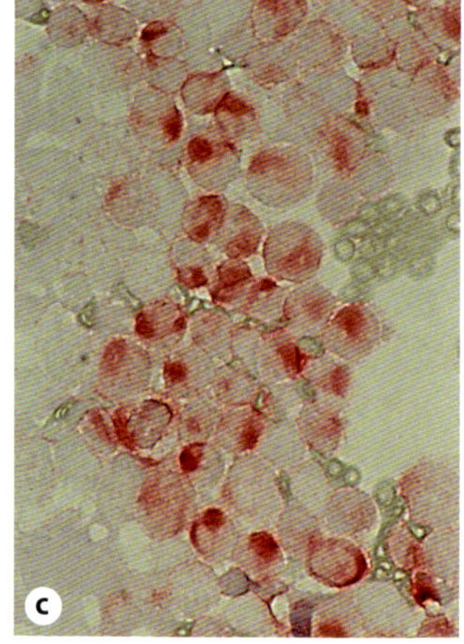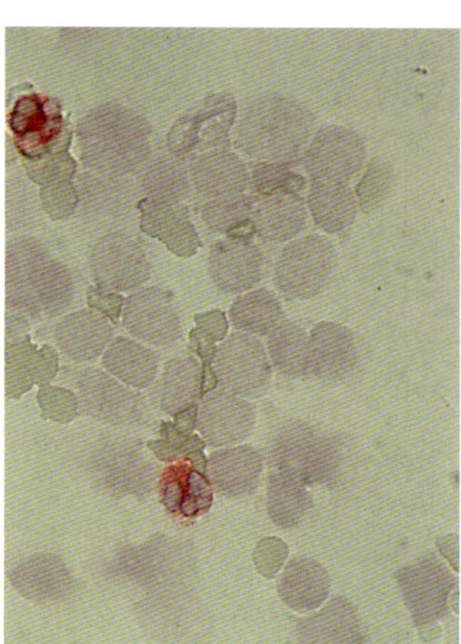

Fig. 10.6. a Merkel cell carcinoma. Clinical presentation showing cutaneous erythematous plaque on the arm. **b** Merkel cell carcinoma. Smear from the aspirate from the skin lesion shown in **a**. The tumor cells are relatively small with scanty cytoplasm and there is a tendency to molding. MGG, high-power view. **c** Merkel cell carcinoma. Immunocytochemistry shows that tumor cells are positive for cytokeratin and negative for CD45. Alkaline phosphatase, high-power view.

Lymphoma-like metastases from malignant melanomas are relatively rare but important to recognize.

Cytologic Features (fig. 10.7a)

The lymphoma look-alike variant of melanoma is composed of a monomorphic tumor cell population of dispersed round cells. The nuclei are round and have a smooth chromatin. The cytoplasm is scanty and melanin is only rarely found, but some vacuoles may be seen. Lymphoglandular bodies are not present [28–31].

Immunocytochemstry (fig. 10.7b): The tumor cells are S-100 and HMB45 positive but lack expression of CD45.

Seminoma/Dysgerminoma

Clinical Features

These tumors occur both in the gonads and in extragonadal localization. The gonadal variant is seen in young adults. It is called seminoma when arising in the testis while the term dys-

germinoma is used for tumors arising in the ovary. Extragonadal tumors are seen in the midline and the most frequent site is the mediastinum but brain and retroperitoneum may also be involved. The symptoms relate to a rapidly growing tumor mass which, depending on the site involved, results in different clinical manifestations. Lymph nodes are the most common site of metastasis but lung, bone and soft tissue can also be affected.

This tumor is highly sensitive to radiation and chemotherapy and the prognosis is good.

Cytology (fig. 10.8a, b)

Most cases have 'classical' cytology with a dispersed population of large round-to-oval cells. The nuclei have an irregular contour and nucleoli are often present.

The cytoplasm is often not visible since the cells are fragile generating a typical 'tigroid' background (fig. 10.8a). Intact cells have an abundant pale, sometimes vacuolated cytoplasm.

There is often an admixture of small lymphocytes and in some cases epitheloid cells and multinucleated giant cells are also present (fig. 10.8b) [32].

Lymphoma Look-Alike

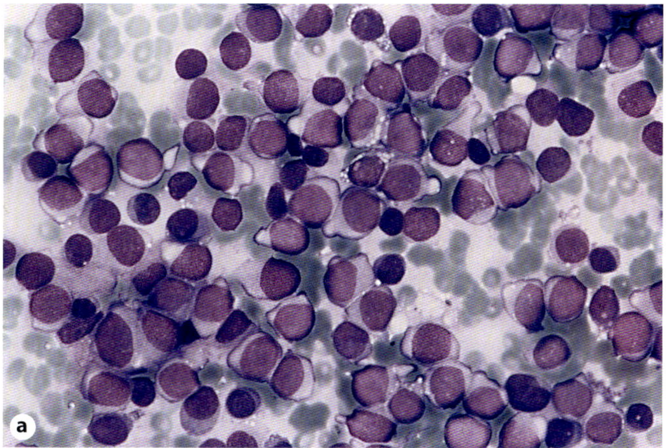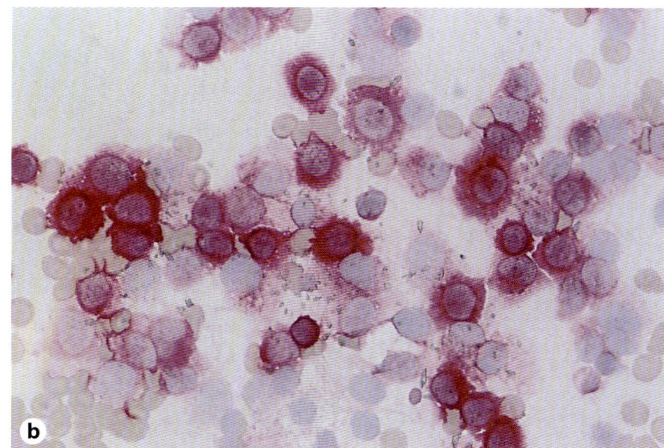

Fig. 10.7. **a** Malignant melanoma. Smear shows a lymphoma look alike variant of melanoma composed of monomorphic dispersed tumor cells with distinct relatively sparse cytoplasm and round nuclei. MGG, high-power view. **b** Malignant melanoma. Immunocytochemistry of the same case as in **a**. The tumor cells are positive for HMB45. Alkaline phosphatase, high-power view.

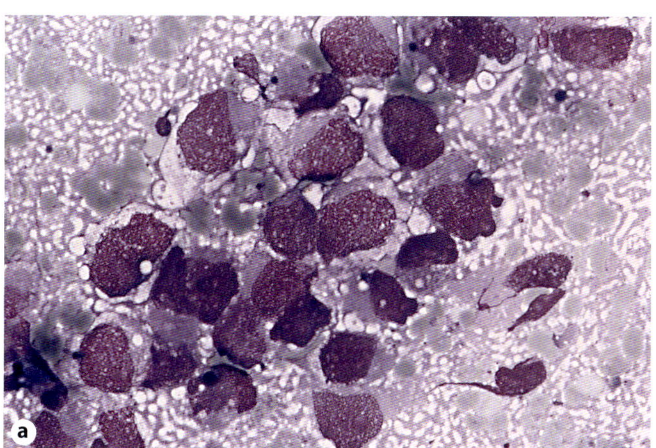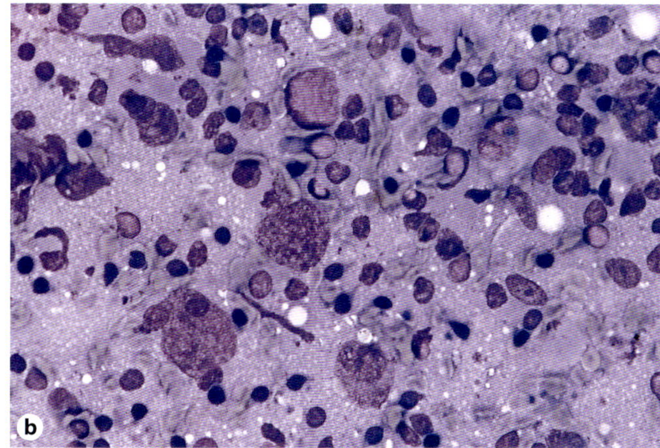

Fig. 10.8. **a** Dysgerminoma. Smear shows large dispersed tumor cells with irregular nuclei with poorly defined grey-blue cytoplasm in a 'tigroid' background. MGG, high-power view. **b** Seminoma. Smear show large dispersed tumor cells admix with small lymphocytes. MGG, high-power view.

The anaplastic variant features large cells showing marked pleomorphism. A conclusive diagnosis of this subtype can only be made after immunophenotyping.

Immunocytochemistry: The cells express PLAP and NSE. Approximately 50% of the cases express vimentin. AFP is negative.

Desmoplastic Round Cell Tumor

Clinical Features

Children and young adults are primarily affected and there is a distinct male predominance [33]. It almost exclusively presents in the abdominal cavity with pain, distension, obstruction and a palpable tumor as the dominating symptoms. It is a highly aggressive tumor with poor survival.

Cytology (fig. 10.9)

Smears show small tumor cells with indistinct, scant cytoplasm. The hyperchromatic nuclei are irregular, oval and vary in size. Mitotic figures are common [34–36]. In addition, collagen fragments and fibroblasts are often found.

Immunocytochemistry: The phenotype is complex and most cells express vimentin, cytokeratin, desmin and NSE [33]. Staining for WT-1 is typically nuclear.

Cytogenetics: All cases show t(22;22) with a fusion of the EWS and WT-1 gene.

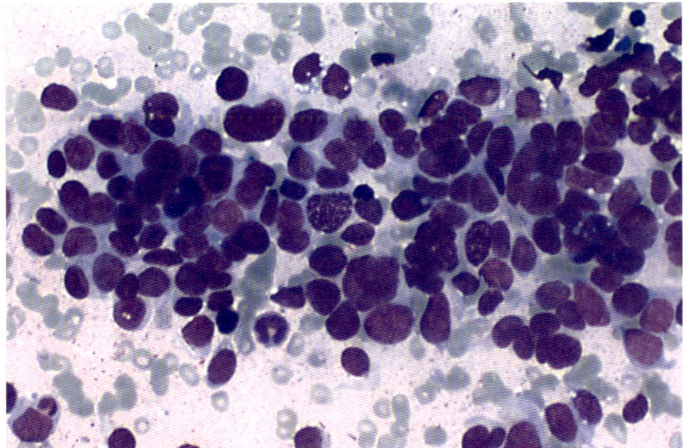

Fig. 10.9. Desmoplastic small round cell tumor. Cluster of loosely attached tumor cells with irregular nuclei of varying size and poorly defined, scanty light blue cytoplasm. MGG, high-power view.

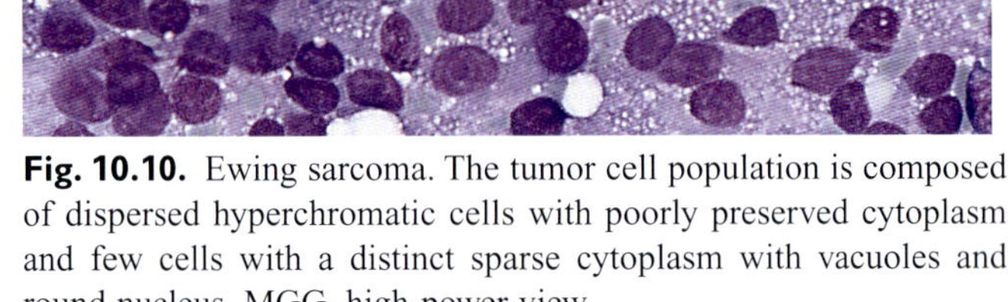

Fig. 10.10. Ewing sarcoma. The tumor cell population is composed of dispersed hyperchromatic cells with poorly preserved cytoplasm and few cells with a distinct sparse cytoplasm with vacuoles and round nucleus. MGG, high-power view.

Childhood Tumors

Aspirates from primary as well as metastatic Ewing's sarcoma, neuroblastoma, rhabdomyosarcoma and Wilms' tumor can sometimes be difficult to differentiate cytologically from lymphoma without immunophenotyping.

Cytology

(1) Smears of aspirates from Ewing's sarcoma (fig. 10.10) usually show two types of cells: one is small with a hyperchromatic nucleus and poorly preserved cytoplasm, and the second cell type is larger with a round nucleus and sparse often vacuolated cytoplasm. Areas with cohesive cells are often present [37–43].

(2) Smears from neuroblastoma (fig. 10.11) show mostly dispersed cells which have a round-to-oval nucleus and sparse cytoplasm. Isolated cells are very difficult to separate from lymphoblasts. In a majority of cases, the cells form rosettes with fibrillar material in the center. This is often easier to find in cytospin preparations. Ganglion-like cells are only found in ganglioneuroblastomas [43–49].

(3) Smears of aspirates of rhabdomyosarcomas of embryonal or alveolar type (fig 10.12) often yield immature round cells with a sparse cytoplasm. There are occasional larger cells with a distinct grey-blue cytoplasm. In the alveolar type, the cells tend to form loose alveolar structures [50–56].

(4) Smears from aspirates of Wilms' tumor (fig. 10.13) can be dominated by immature cells with oval-to-round nuclei and a poorly preserved cytoplasm. Epithelial structures can be identified in most cases [57–61].

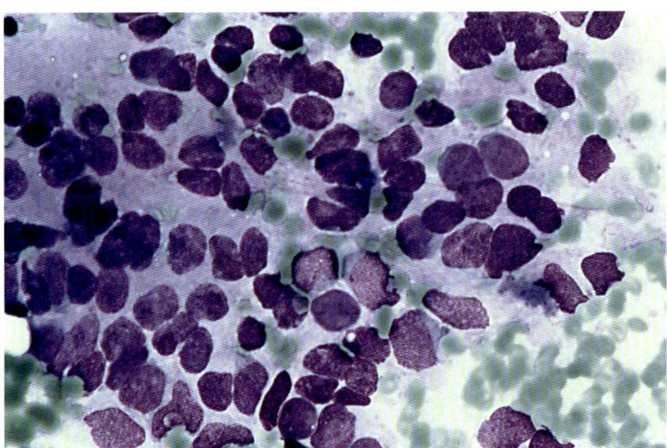

Fig. 10.11. Neuroblastoma. Smear shows few tumor cells with round nuclei and scant rim of pale blue cytoplasm. The dominating cells have irregular nuclear form with tendency to form rosettes (upper left) and indistinct cytoplasm. MGG, high-power view.

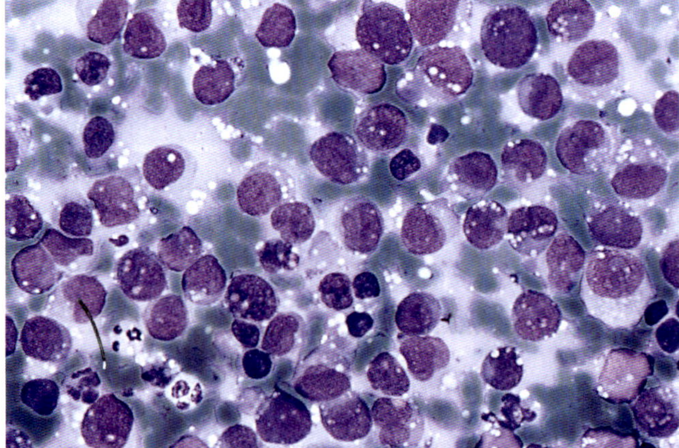

Fig. 10.12. Rhabdomyosarcoma, alveolar type. Smear shows dispersed immature round cells with sparse distinct cytoplasm with vacuoles. MGG, high-power view.

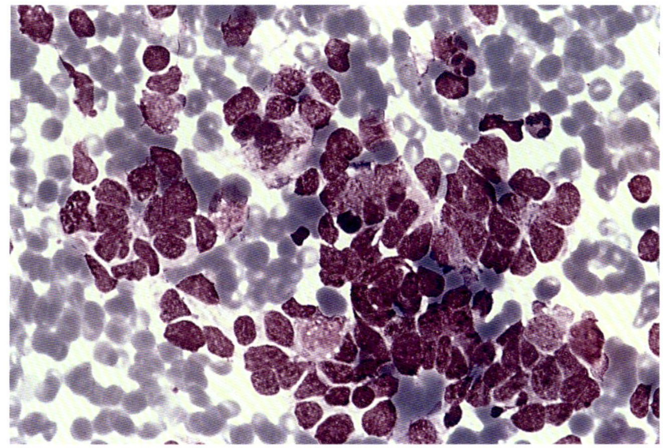

Fig. 10.13. Wilms' tumor. Smear shows clusters of immature cells with irregular nuclei and indistinct cytoplasm. MGG, high-power view.

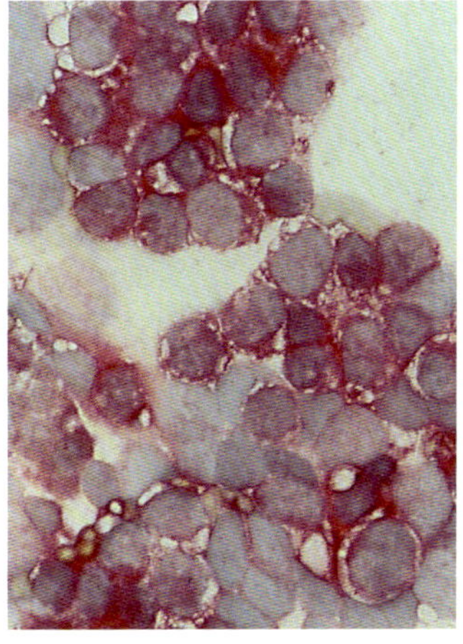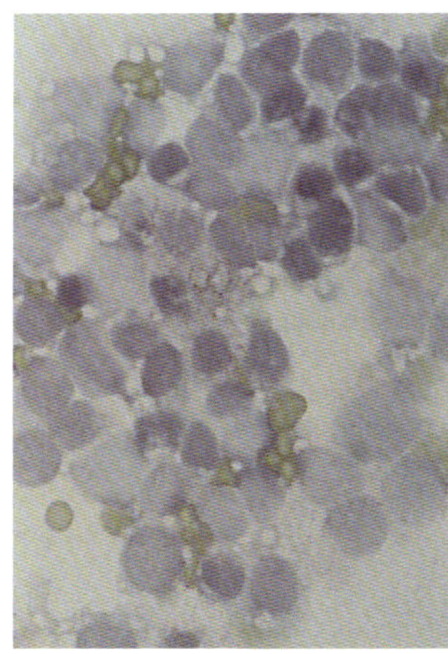

Fig. 10.14. Ewing sarcoma. Tumor cells are CD99+ (left) and CD45− (right) . Alkaline phosphate, high-power view.

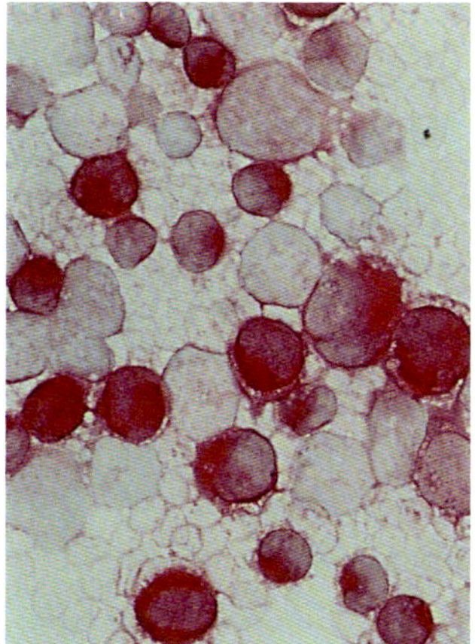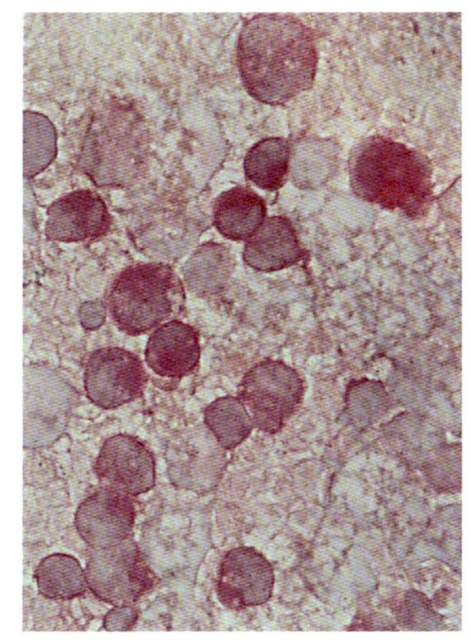

Fig. 10.15. Rhabdomyosarcoma, alveolar type. The cells are desmin (left) and myoglobulin positive (right). Alkaline phosphatase, high-power view.

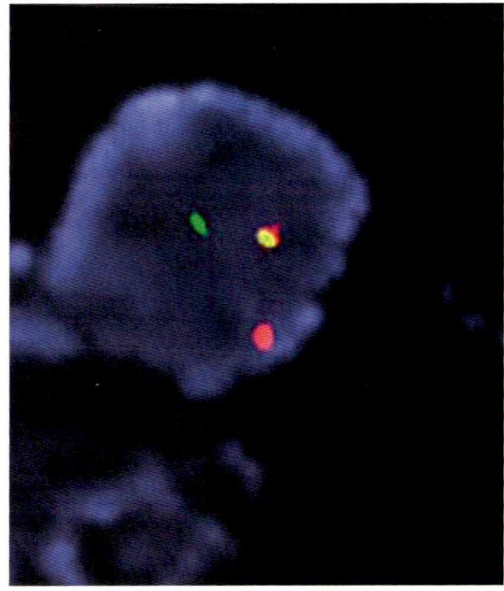

Fig. 10.16. Ewing sarcoma. Interphase FISH on tumor cells using Vysis LSI EWSRI (22q12) Dual Color, Break Apart Rearrangement Prove. In the tumor cell, a rearrangement of the EWS gene splits the green and red signal apart. These signals are fused in a normal cell. Courtesy of Dr. E. Blennow, Clinical Genetics, Karolinska University Hospital.

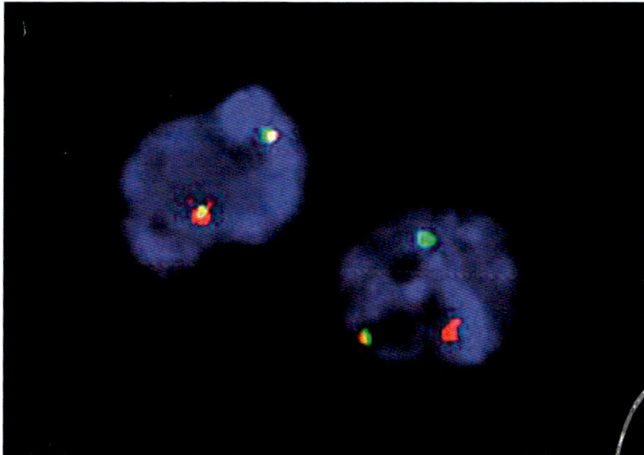

Fig. 10.17. Rhabdomyosarcoma. Interphase FISH on tumor cells using Vysis LSI FKHR (13q14) Dual Color, Break Apart Rearrangement Probe. A normal cell (left) shows two fusion signals, while rearrangement of FKHR in the tumor cell (right) splits the red and green signal apart. Courtesy of Dr. E. Blennow, Clinical Genetics, Karolinska University Hospital Solna, Stockholm.

Immunocytochemistry: Ewing's sarcoma cells are vimentin, CD99 and NSE positive (fig. 10.14). Neuroblastoma cells are N84 and NSE positive. Rhabdomyosarcoma cells are vimentin, desmin, actin and myoglobulin positive (fig. 10.15). Wilms' tumor cells express vimentin and WT-1.

Cytogenetics: Ewing's sarcoma cells present translocation t(11;22) (fig. 10.16), while rhabdomyosarcomas of the alveolar type typically show translocation t(2;13) (fig. 10.17).

References

1 Das D: Lymph nodes; in Bibbo M (ed): Comprehensive Cytopathology, ed 2. Philadelphia, Saunders, 1997, pp 703–731.

2 Orell S, Sterrett G, Walters M, Whitaker D, van Heerde P: Lymph nodes; in Orell S, Sterrett G, Walters M, Whitaker D (eds): Fine Needle Aspiration Cytology, ed 4. London, Churchill-Livingstone, 2005, pp 74–108.

3 Kocjan G: Lymph nodes; in Kocjan G (ed): Clinical Cytopathology of the Head and Neck. London, Greenwich Medical Media, 2001.

4 Skoog L, Tani E: Lymph nodes; in Gray W, McKee GT (eds): Diagnostic Cytopathology, ed 2. Hong Kong, Churchill-Livingstone, 2003, pp 492–503.

5 Caraway NP, Katz RL: Lymph nodes; in Koss LG, Melamed MR (eds): Koss' Diagnostic Cytology and Its Histopathologic Bases, ed 5. Philadelphia, Lippincott Williams & Wilkins, 2006, pp 1186–1228.

6 Shabb N, Katz R, Ordonez N, Goodacre A, Hirsch-Ginsberg C, el-Naggar A: Fine-needle aspiration evaluation of lymphoproliferative lesions in human immunodeficiency virus-positive patients: a multiparameter approach. Cancer 1991;67:1008–1018.

7 Prasad RR, Narasimhan R, Sankaran V, Veliath AJ: Fine-needle aspiration cytology in the diagnosis of superficial lymphadenopathy: an analysis of 2,418 cases. Diagn Cytopathol 1996;15:382–386.

8 Kardos TF, Kornstein MJ, Frable WJ: Cytology and immunocytology of infectious mononucleosis in fine needle aspirates of lymph nodes. Acta Cytol 1988;32:722–726.

9 Stanley MW, Steeper TA, Horwitz CA, Burton LG, Strickler JG, Borken S: Fine-needle aspiration of lymph nodes in patients with acute infectious mononucleosis. Diagn Cytopathol 1990;6:323–329.

10 Pettinato G, Manivel JC, d'Amore ES, Petrella G: Fine needle aspiration cytology and immunocytochemical characterization of the histiocytes in sinus histiocytosis with massive lymphadenopathy (Rosai-Dorfman syndrome). Acta Cytol 1990;34:771

11 Schmitt FC: Sinus histiocytosis with massive lymphadenopathy (Rosai-Dorfman disease): cytomorphologic analysis on fine-needle aspirates. Diagn Cytopathol 1992;8:586.

12 Stastny JF, Wilkerson ML, Hamati HF, Kornstein MJ: Cytologic features of sinus hisitiocytosis with massive lymphadenopathy: a report of three cases. Acta Cytol 1997;41:871–876.

13 Deshpande V, Verma K: Fine needle aspiration (FNA) cytology of Rosai-Dorfman disease. Cytopathology 1998;9:329.

14 Das DK, Gulati A, Bhatt NC, Sethi GR: Sinus histiocytosis with massive lymphadenopathy (Rosai-dorfman disease): report of two cases with fine-needle aspiration cytology. Diagn Cytopathol 2001;24:42–45.

15 Verma K, Rao AV, Kapila K: Cytologic diagnosis of an acute myeloid leukemia infiltrate in a lymph node. Acta Cytol 1991;35:373–374.

16 Bangerter M, Hildebrand A, Waidmann O, Griesshammer M: Diagnosis of granulocytic sarcoma by fine needle aspiration cytology. Acta Haematol 2000;103:102–108.

17 Kumar PV, Karimi M, Monabati A, Sadeghipour AR, Tavangar SM, Moosavi A, Nourani H, Haghkshanas M, Bedayat GR: Cytology of leukemic lymphadenopathy. Acta Cytol 2002;46:801–807.

18 Scarpa C, Trevisan G, Stinco G: Lyme borreliosis. Dermatol Clin 1994;12:669–685.

19 Liu YJ, Lee YT, Hsieh SW, Kuo SH: Presumption of primary sites of neck lymph node metastases on fine needle aspiration cytology. Acta Cytol 1997;41:1477–1482.

20 Kollur SM, El Hag IA: Fine-needle aspiration cytology of metastatic nasopharyngeal carcinoma in cervical lymph nodes: comparison with metastatic squamous-cell carcinoma, and Hodgkin's and non-Hodgkin's lymphoma. Diagn Cytopathol 2003;28:18–22.

21 De Las Casas LE, Gokden M, Mukunyadzi P, White P, Baker SJ, Hermonat PL, You H, Korourian S, Malak SF, Miranda RN: A morphologic and statistical comparative study of small-cell carcinoma and non-Hodgkin's lymphoma in fine-needle aspiration biopsy material from lymph nodes. Diagn Cytopathol 2004;31:229–234.

22 Shin HJ, Caraway NP: Fine needle biopsy of Metastatic small cell carcinoma from extrapulmonary sites. Diagn. Cytopathol 1998;19:177–181.

23 Skoog L, Schmitt FC, Tani E: Neuroendocrine (Merkel cell) carcinoma of the skin: immunocytochemical and cytomorphological analysis on fine needle aspirates. Diagn Cytopathol 1990;6:53–57.

24 Layfield LJ, Glasgow BJ: Aspiration biopsy cytology of primary cutaneous tumors. Acta Cytol 1993;37:679–688.

25 Collins BT, Elmberger PG, Tani EM, Bjornhagen V, Ramos RR: Fine-needle aspiration of Merkel cell carcinoma of the skin with cytomorphology and immunocytochemical correlation. Diagn Cytopathol 1998;18:251–257.

26 Dey P, Jogai S, Amir T, Temim L: Fine-needle aspiration cytology of Merkel cell carcinoma. Diagn Cytopathol 2004;31:364–365.

27 Daugherty HK Jr, Rumboldt T, Hoda RS: Contralateral metastasis of a cutaneous Merkel cell carcinoma: diagnosis by fine needle aspiration cytology. Diagn Cytopathol 2005;33:450–451.

28 Kapila K, Kharbanda K, Verma K: Cytomorphology of metastatic melanoma – use of S-100 protein in the diagnosis of amelanotic melanoma. Cytopathology 1991;2:229–237.

29 Nasiell K, Tani E, Skoog L: Fine needle aspiration cytology and immunocytochemistry of metastatic melanoma. Cytopathology 1991;2:137–147.

30 Simmons TJ, Martin SE: Fine-needle aspiration biopsy of malignant melanoma: a cytologic and immunocytochemical analysis. Diagn Cytopathol 1991;7:380–386.

31 Saqi A, McGrath CM, Skovronsky D, Yu GH: Cytomorphologic features of fine-needle aspiration of metastatic and recurrent melanoma. Diagn Cytopathol 2002;27:286–290.

32 Fleury-Feith J, Bellot-Besnard J: Criteria for aspiration cytology for the diagnosis of seminoma. Diagn Cytopathol 1989;5:392–395.

33 Antonescu CR, Gerald W: Desmoplastic small round cell tumor; in Fletcher DM, Unni KK, Merteus F (eds): Tumours of Soft Tissue and Bone. Geneva, WHO, 2002, pp 216–218.

34 Akthar M, Ali MA, Sabbah R, et al: Small round cell tumor with divergent differentiation: cytologic, histologic and ultrastructural findings. Diagn Cytopathol 1994;11:159–164.

35 Ferlicot S, Cové O, Gilbert E, et al: Intraabdominal desmoplastic small round cell tumor: report a case with fine needle aspiration, cytologic diagnosis and molecular conformation. Acta Cytol 2001;45:617–621

36 Dave B, Shet T, Chinoy R: Desmoplastic round cell tumor of childhood: can cytology with immunocytochemistry serve as an alternative for tissue diagnosis. Diagn Cytopathol 2005;32:330–335.

37 Mondal A, Misra DK: Ewing's sarcoma of bone: a study of 71 cases by fine needle aspiration cytology. J Indian Med Assoc 1996;94:135–137, 142.

38 Collins BT, Cramer HM, Frain BE, Davis MM: Fine-needle aspiration biopsy of metastatic Ewing's sarcoma with MIC2 (CD99) immunocytochemistry. Diagn Cytopathol 1998;19:382–384.

39 Sahu K, Pai RR, Khadilkar UN: Fine needle aspiration cytology of the Ewing's sarcoma family of tumors. Acta Cytol 2000;44:332–336.

40 Agarwal S, Agarwal T, Agarwal R, Agarwal PK, Jain UK: Fine needle aspiration of bone tumors. Cancer Detect Prev 2000;24:602–609.

41 Brahmi U, Rajwanshi A, Joshi K, Ganguly NK, Vohra H, Gupta SK, Dey P: Role of immunocytochemistry and DNA flow cytometry in the fine-needle aspiration diagnosis of malignant small round-cell tumors. Diagn Cytopathol 2001;24:233–239.

42 Frostad B, Tani E, Brosjo O, Skoog L, Kogner P: Fine needle aspiration cytology in the diagnosis and management of children and adolescents with Ewing sarcoma and peripheral primitive neuroectodermal tumor. Med Pediatr Oncol 2002;38:33–40.

43 Brahmi U, Rajwanshi A, Joshi K, Ganguly NK, Vohra H, Gupta SK, Dey P: Role of immunocytochemistry and DNA flow cytometry in the fine-needle aspiration diagnosis of malignant small round-cell tumors. Diagn Cytopathol 2001;24:233–239.

44 Akhtar M, Iqbal MA, Mourad W, Ali MA: Fine-needle aspiration biopsy diagnosis of small round cell tumors of childhood: a comprehensive approach. Diagn Cytopathol 1999;21:81–91.

45 Das DK: Fine-needle aspiration (FNA) cytology diagnosis of small round cell tumors: value and limitations. Indian J Pathol Microbiol 2004;47:309–318.

46 Drut R, Drut RM, Pollono D, Tomarchio S, Ibanez O, Urrutia A, Ripoll MC: Fine-needle aspiration biopsy in pediatric oncology patients: a review of experience with 829 patients (899 biopsies). J Pediatr Hematol Oncol 2005;27:370–376.

47 Das DK, Bhambhani S, Chachra KL, Murthy NS, Tripathi RP: Small round cell tumors of the abdomen and thorax: role of fine needle aspiration cytologic features in the diagnosis and differential diagnosis. Acta Cytol 1997;41:1035–1047.

48 Fröstad B, Tani E, Kogner P, Maeda S, Björk O, Skoog L: The clinical use of fine needle aspiration cytology for diagnosis and management of children with neuroblastic tumours. Eur J Cancer 1998;34:529–536.

49 Thiesse P, Hany MA, Combaret V, Ranchere-Vince D, Bouffet E, Bergeron C: Assessment of percutaneous fine needle aspiration cytology as a technique to provide diagnostic and prognostic information in neuroblastoma. Eur J Cancer. 2000;36:1544–1551.

50 Akhtar M, Ali MA, Bakry M, Hug M, Sackey K: Fine-needle aspiration biopsy diagnosis of rhabdomyosarcoma: cytologic, histologic, and ultrastructural correlations. Diagn Cytopathol 1992;8:465–474.

51 de Almeida M, Stastny JF, Wakely PE Jr, Frable WJ: Fine-needle aspiration biopsy of childhood rhabdomyosarcoma: reevaluation of the cytologic criteria for diagnosis. Diagn Cytopathol 1994;11:231–236.

52 Atahan S, Aksu O, Ekinci C: Cytologic diagnosis and subtyping of rhabdomyosarcoma. Cytopathology 1998;9:389–397.

53 Pohar-Marinsek Z, Anzic J, Jereb B: Topical topic: value of fine needle aspiration biopsy in childhood rhabdomyosarcoma: twenty-six years of experience in Slovenia. Med Pediatr Oncol 2002;38:416–420.

54 Pohar-Marinsek Z, Bracko M: Rhabdomyosarcoma. Cytomorphology, subtyping and differential diagnostic dilemmas. Acta Cytol 2000;44:524–532.

55 Pohar-Marinsek Z, Anzic J, Jereb B: Topical topic: value of fine needle aspiration biopsy in childhood rhabdomyosarcoma: twenty-six years of experience in Slovenia. Med Pediatr Oncol 2002;38:416–420.

56 Chen KT: Rhabdomyosarcoma in an adult presenting with nodal metastasis: a pitfall infine-needle aspiration cytology of lymph nodes. Diagn Cytopathol 2005;32:303–306.

57 Dey P, Radhika S, Rajwanshi A, Rao KL, Khajuria A, Nijhawan R, Banarjee CK: Aspiration cytology of Wilms' tumor. Acta Cytol 1993;37:477–482.

58 Hazarika D, Narasimhamurthy KN, Rao CR, Gopinath KS: Fine needle aspiration cytology of Wilms' tumor: a study of 17 cases. Acta Cytol 1994;38:355–360.

59 Iyer VK, Kapila K, Agarwala S, Dinda AK, Verma K: Wilms' tumor. Role of fine needle aspiration and DNA ploidy by image analysis in prognostication. Anal Quant Cytol Histol 1999;21:505–511.

60 Li P, Perle MA, Scholes JV, Yang GC: Wilms' tumor in adults: aspiration cytology and cytogenetics. Diagn Cytopathol 2002;26:99–103.

61 Ravindra S, Kini U: Cytomorphology and morphometry of small round-cell tumors in the region of the kidney. Diagn Cytopathol 2005;32:211–216.

Index

  Index